Coping

Dr Sallie Baxendale is a consultant clinical neuropsy... has worked with people with memory difficulties in the NHS fo... ...nty years. She is the author of over fifty academic publications ... ...ory function. Her work in this field ranges from the development o... ...hab-ilitation strategies to studies of the ways in which memory problems are misrepresented in the media. She currently works for the Institute of Neurology, University College London.

Overcoming Common Problems Series

Selected titles

A full list of titles is available from Sheldon Press,
36 Causton Street, London SW1P 4ST and on our website at
www.sheldonpress.co.uk

101 Questions to Ask Your Doctor
Dr Tom Smith

Asperger Syndrome in Adults
Dr Ruth Searle

Assertiveness: Step by step
Dr Windy Dryden and Daniel Constantinou

Birth Over 35
Sheila Kitzinger

Body Language: What you need to know
David Cohen

Breast Cancer: Your treatment choices
Dr Terry Priestman

Bulimia, Binge-eating and their Treatment
Professor J. Hubert Lacey, Dr Bryony Bamford
and Amy Brown

The Cancer Survivor's Handbook
Dr Terry Priestman

The Chronic Pain Diet Book
Neville Shone

Cider Vinegar
Margaret Hills

Coeliac Disease: What you need to know
Alex Gazzola

**Coping Successfully with Chronic Illness:
Your healing plan**
Neville Shone

Coping Successfully with Pain
Neville Shone

Coping Successfully with Prostate Cancer
Dr Tom Smith

Coping Successfully with Shyness
Margaret Oakes, Professor Robert Bor
and Dr Carina Eriksen

Coping Successfully with Ulcerative Colitis
Peter Cartwright

Coping Successfully with Varicose Veins
Christine Craggs-Hinton

Coping Successfully with Your Hiatus Hernia
Dr Tom Smith

Coping When Your Child Has Cerebral Palsy
Jill Eckersley

Coping with Anaemia
Dr Tom Smith

Coping with Asthma in Adults
Mark Greener

**Coping with Birth Trauma and Postnatal
Depression**
Lucy Jolin

Coping with Bronchitis and Emphysema
Dr Tom Smith

Coping with Candida
Shirley Trickett

Coping with Chemotherapy
Dr Terry Priestman

Coping with Chronic Fatigue
Trudie Chalder

Coping with Difficult Families
Dr Jane McGregor and Tim McGregor

Coping with Diverticulitis
Peter Cartwright

Coping with Drug Problems in the Family
Lucy Jolin

Coping with Dyspraxia
Jill Eckersley

Coping with Early-onset Dementia
Jill Eckersley

Coping with Eating Disorders and Body Image
Christine Craggs-Hinton

Coping with Epilepsy
Dr Pamela Crawford and Fiona Marshall

Coping with Gout
Christine Craggs-Hinton

Coping with Guilt
Dr Windy Dryden

Coping with Headaches and Migraine
Alison Frith

Coping with Heartburn and Reflux
Dr Tom Smith

Coping with Life after Stroke
Dr Mareeni Raymond

**Coping with Life's Challenges: Moving on
from adversity**
Dr Windy Dryden

Coping with Liver Disease
Mark Greener

Overcoming Common Problems Series

Overcoming Common Problems Series

Overcoming Common Problems

Coping with Memory Problems

DR SALLIE BAXENDALE

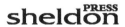

First published in Great Britain in 2014

Sheldon Press
36 Causton Street
London SW1P 4ST
www.sheldonpress.co.uk

British Library Cataloguing-in-Publication Data
A catalogue record for this book is available from the British Library

ISBN 978-1-84709-274-8
eBook ISBN 978-1-84709-275-5

Typeset by Fakenham Prepress Solutions, Fakenham, Norfolk NR21 8NN
First printed in Great Britain by Ashford Colour Press
Subsequently digitally reprinted in Great Britain

eBook by Fakenham Prepress Solutions, Fakenham, Norfolk NR21 8NN

Produced on paper from sustainable forests

For Jane,
the best of friends
and the very best memories

Contents

1

Introduction

You'd forget your head if it wasn't screwed on.

I've got the memory of a goldfish.

My memory's a sieve.

Memory lapses are such a part of everyday life that the English language is peppered with clichés to describe them. They are almost as much a feature of British conversation as the weather. When people share their embarrassing anecdotes about a failure to recognize a work colleague in the street, or describe the convoluted steps they had to take to avoid using the elusive name of an acquaintance in a chance encounter, they are almost always met with the reply, 'Oh I know . . . The same thing happened to me this morning/yesterday/last week.' And so these tales of memory difficulties appear to be universal and, perhaps, nothing to worry about. But for some people, these memory lapses happen too often and the resulting consequences are too problematic and embarrassing for them to just be dismissed as part of everyday life.

Confiding in close friends can often make us feel better about our problems. Even if there aren't any practical solutions to be had, we can usually derive a great deal of comfort from the feeling that somebody understands and empathizes with our situation. But when people try to express their concerns about memory problems, the frequent response of 'Oh that happens to me all the time' can leave them feeling even more isolated and anxious than before. You may suspect that your memory lapses are out of the ordinary, but getting other people to understand the worrisome extent of the problem can be very difficult indeed. When you are left to your own devices, all kinds of terrifying thoughts may run through your mind as to why your memory might be going downhill, with the frightening spectre of dementia often hovering on the horizon. Some people may find that they slowly withdraw from friends

1

and family members as they lose confidence in their ability to remember and discuss past events, further increasing their isolation. The resulting anxiety, low mood and depression this generates often exacerbates the original memory difficulties and so a downward spiral of deterioration begins.

If you are struggling with memory problems yourself or are caring for someone who has memory difficulties, this book has been written to help you cope. It is divided into two sections. The first half of the book explains how memory works. Once you understand how something works, it's easier to see where and why the process may be breaking down and, if it is broken, how it might be fixed. Although people will often use the blanket phrase 'my memory is terrible' the brain uses many different mechanisms to store and retrieve information and, even in people with far-reaching memory difficulties, not all systems are affected to the same extent. Each chapter in the first part of this book describes a different aspect of memory. Chapter 2 explains the importance of paying attention to new information in the first place. It may sound obvious, but if you have not paid attention to something, you have no hope of remembering it later. This failure to attend to new information underlies many common memory complaints. Chapter 3 debunks some of the common myths about memory and explains why it is not surprising at all that you can remember events from your childhood with Blu-ray-like clarity, while what you did last Wednesday is swathed in an impenetrable peasouper of a brain fog. Chapter 4 explains why you never forget how to ride a bike, while Chapter 5 looks to the future and explains how we remember the things we need to do and the places we need to be every day. It's all about remembering to remember. Chapter 6 examines the ways we retrieve information from our long-term memory store and looks at some of the things that can get in the way and block this process. It's a lot to do with the way that the information was stored in the first place. This chapter also examines one of the most frustrating and ubiquitous memory complaints we hear in the memory clinic: word-finding difficulties or the 'tip of the tongue' phenomenon.

Chapters 2 to 6 explain how these separate memory systems work and describe strategies that you can use to boost your brain power and reduce the nuisance that failures in each area can cause in everyday life.

The second half of the book looks at some of the most common underlying causes of memory problems.

Throughout the book, reference is made to the hippocampi (plural). The word is taken from the Greek word for 'seahorses'. The hippocampi are two seahorse-shaped structures in the brain that play a crucial role in creating new memories. There is one on the right-hand side and one on the left-hand side of the brain. It is still possible to form new memories if one hippocampus is damaged, but if both are damaged severe memory problems occur. Generally speaking, large, plump hippocampi are an indication of a healthy memory system. However, there are many factors that have a detrimental impact on hippocampal health and that cause the structures to shrink. The second half of the book examines some of these factors and ways in which you can ensure your hippocampi stay as healthy as possible.

Mood, physical health and hormonal changes can all have a very significant impact on memory function. Chapters 8 to 12 explain these effects. It is well known that diet and exercise have a significant impact on physical health. More and more research now supports the fact that they have a significant impact on cognitive ageing too. A healthy diet and regular moderate exercise in middle age are associated with reduced odds of developing a progressive memory impairment in old age. Even in old age, when there are physical changes within the brain and some hippocampal shrinkage is inevitable, regular physical exercise can slow down and even reverse some of these changes. Chapter 10 describes some of the ways that you can maximize the health of your hippocampi. It's never too late to make beneficial lifestyle changes. Similarly, keeping mentally active may also help to keep memory problems at bay. Chapter 12 describes some of the exciting new research that suggests that the 'use it or lose it' rule applies to cognitive functions, just as it does to muscles.

Everybody's memory starts to decline as we get older. While scientific studies have shown that some of our cognitive abilities start to deteriorate from our mid-twenties (!), it is often in middle age that people really begin to notice that their memory is not what it was. It can be difficult to know what is within the bounds of normality and what isn't. Chapter 12 explains the patterns that are expected in normal ageing.

For some people memory problems are a symptom of something more serious than just normal ageing or increased stress. Chapter 14, 'When to seek further help', describes some of the tell-tale signs that something more than just normal age-related decline may be responsible for the memory problems you or your loved one experiences, and offers some advice about when it may be appropriate to seek help and support from your GP.

There are no silver bullets when it comes to improving memory function. This, as you will see, is a recurrent theme throughout the book. The strategies that can be used to cope with memory problems can be broadly divided into three groups:

1 those that deal with the underlying problem;
2 internal strategies that you can use to exploit the way your brain works;
3 outsourcing your memory functions to external agencies to reduce the load.

The first group of strategies tackles underlying problems that are interfering with memory processing. There is a surprising amount that you can do, even if your underlying brain systems are damaged, to maximize your efficiency in this regard (see Chapters 8 to 11). The second set of strategies focuses on ways in which you can get the most out of your memory to try to maximize the likelihood that new information goes in and is properly processed in the first place, and minimize the obstacles that might prevent you from recalling it fluently later. The final group of strategies involves taking the load off an overburdened memory system by using external aids (from the good old-fashioned calendar to the most complex interactive digital apps) to record your information and jog your memory for you. This three-pronged approach is unlikely to solve all your memory problems but it may go a long way to reducing the nuisance they cause in everyday life, and that reduction lies at the heart of coping with memory difficulties.

Part 1
HOW MEMORY WORKS

2

Are you paying attention?
Then we will begin . . .

There is a very famous psychology experiment involving basketball players and a man in a gorilla suit. In the experiment, students were asked to watch a video of people throwing a ball to each other and were told to count the number of times the ball is passed from one player to another. There are two balls in play, so viewers have to concentrate reasonably hard to ensure that they don't get distracted by the other ball being passed around by a different team. At the end of the video the students were asked two questions.

1 How many times was the ball passed?
2 Did you see the dancing gorilla?

Halfway through the film, a man in a gorilla suit walks plainly into the centre of the scene, stops to do a little dance, centre-stage, and then ambles slowly off again. This is not a subliminal image, flashed on the screen for a few micro seconds. It is an unmissable part of the film. And yet 40 per cent of the students who watched the video completely failed to spot the gorilla. While their attention was so entirely taken up with counting the number of ball passes, they just didn't process the information that was clearly on the screen they were so intently looking at.

In the second phase of the study, about one third of the students who took part had heard about the study beforehand. They knew a gorilla was going to appear at some point and were ready and waiting. In addition to counting the ball passes they kept an eye out for the gorilla and easily spotted him meandering across the stage. However, even though they knew about the nature of the experiment, a significant number of these students failed to notice that one of the players left the game halfway through and that the background to the scene completely changed colour.

In another famous study, the experimenters were manning a reception desk. Whenever a new customer came to the desk and asked for information the 'receptionist' (who was actually one of the experimenters) would chat a while and then duck under the desk, ostensibly to retrieve a relevant information leaflet. Immediately afterwards an entirely different person (who had been hiding under the desk) popped back up with the leaflet and continued the conversation with the unsuspecting customer. Again, about half of the customers who unwittingly took part in this experiment failed to notice that the receptionist had changed.

This phenomenon isn't just limited to psychology experiments. It happens in everyday life too. In 2008, a family home in Manchester was burgled early on a Saturday evening. Not that unusual perhaps, except that the burglar stole items from the room in which the whole family sat watching a talent show on the television. Every member of the family was so engrossed by the programme that they all failed to notice someone coming into the room, taking their stuff and leaving with it. YouTube contains a clip, viewed over a million times, of a young man playing 'Minecraft', a popular, addictive computer game. While he is playing the game his house is being burgled, but the young man is so focused on his computer game that he doesn't respond to the obvious sounds of the break-in for some time.

The psychology studies and these anecdotal stories tell us a lot about how we process information. It's tempting to think of our eyes, ears and brain as a kind of video camera, capturing everything we're exposed to in an objective, all-inclusive fashion. But in fact, everything we 'see' has already been filtered and edited by our brains, long before we consciously process the new information. All too often we see what we expect to see and just don't notice the other stuff going on around us. We have evolved this way for a purpose.

Take a moment now to really focus on your environment. Up until this moment you have (hopefully) been concentrating on reading this book. But listen. What can you hear? Chances are you will become aware of something that you were not aware of before, maybe a clock ticking or traffic noise, a computer whirring, or even the sound of your own breathing. Can you smell anything? These noises and smells were there before, but you were not conscious of them because you were focused on reading this book. Without this in-built filter, it is extremely hard to concentrate on anything. Everything distracts us from everything else. In 2011, neuroscientists in Canada coined the term 'bouncer brain cells' to describe the neurons that appear to decide what information they should let into our brains. They recorded the cells 'lighting up' in the front part of the brain, as the bouncers blocked irrelevant information in an experimental task. If this part of the brain is damaged or the bouncer cells don't perform properly for one reason or another, each new element in our environment is given equal importance, and the brain soon becomes overwhelmed. Doctors believe that problems with these neurons could be the source of some of the symptoms of conditions like attention deficit disorder and schizophrenia. And so, without us even being aware of it, our brains filter out the irrelevant stimuli in our environment and help us to focus on whatever we have prioritized for the moment.

This is the first stage in the memory process. To remember something, we have to have paid proper attention to it in the first place. When we are in an environment with several different things competing for our attention, the bouncer cells sometimes make a wrong call and we miss the important information. Even in a calm, quiet environment, we can be distracted by our own thoughts. There is then no chance of retrieving something from our memory if it never got there in the first place. This may seem obvious, but a failure to attend to something in the first place underlies many of the most common memory problems that people experience.

My colleague introduced his wife at the party and just 30 seconds later I just couldn't remember her name at all – it was so awkward.

I used to love reading, but now I just find that I get to the end of the page and have no memory at all of what I've just read. So I find myself reading and re-reading the same page over and over again. It's so frustrating.

I get back to the car park and just can't remember where I parked the car. Sometimes I just have to walk through the rows systematically until I spot it. It's so embarrassing, just wandering around a car park, pressing the remote control keys hoping that the car will beep so I can find it.

> I was halfway to work when I just had to turn back, I just couldn't remember if I had turned the iron off or not. I was late for work, it was so annoying.

Frustrating, embarrassing, annoying, awkward – these common 'memory' failures frequently generate all these feelings. But often we haven't given ourselves a chance in these situations. The information just hasn't been processed properly in the first place. Take the all too common failure to remember the name of someone you have only just been introduced to. When we meet someone for the first time there is usually a lot going on. It's often in a busy social situation and there may be many new and unfamiliar faces around, with a high level of background chatter. When you are introduced to someone new, you will probably be concentrating on the person's face, noticing all kinds of things about his or her appearance and style of dress, and you will also be monitoring your own actions to ensure the introduction goes smoothly. It is extremely easy for the brain to miss the all-important name of the person while all this is going on. The name just hasn't been processed properly. If this happens to you often, there is a relatively easy way around the awkwardness of spending the next ten minutes trying to find ever more inventive ways of addressing your new acquaintance without using a name. If you know you are about to be introduced to someone, consciously anticipate that you are about to be given his or her name. Be waiting for it. Then interrupt the introducer *as soon as you hear the new name* and use it. If somebody says, 'This is my wife, Jane,' don't let him go on to introduce the other people in the group, but shake Jane's hand, and say, 'Hello, Jane'; if you can say something meaningful about the name (without coming across as creepy!) all the better. This way, you have processed the name by saying it out loud while looking at the person. If the name has some personal connotations that you can't politely share with the group (perhaps she looks like a plain Jane) but that might help you to remember it, it's worth trying to make some connection just in your head. The more deeply you process the information and the more connections you make, the more likely you will be to remember the name later on.

The same principle applies to the common problem of failing to remember whether you have done an everyday task, such as locking the front door or turning off an appliance. Often the reason we can't remember doing these things is that they are so automatic, we weren't really paying attention at the time. Many people are able to multitask with ease. This means that it's easy to turn off the iron, on the way to answering the front door, while replying to a text. The reason we can do all these things at the same time is because some of these tasks are so automatic they don't really require us to consciously attend to them at all. And so the iron gets turned off without us ever really paying the action any attention. It's no surprise, then, that when we come to trying to remember whether we did, in fact, turn off the iron we have no recollection of it. Again, there is a relatively simple solution to these kinds of memory difficulties and again it involves speaking. If, when you turn off the iron, you say *out loud*, 'It is Tuesday morning and I have turned off the iron', you should have little difficulty remembering the action a few hours later. It is important to say it out loud as this ensures that you pay sufficient attention while you are completing the action for it to be consciously registered. Also you need to make it time specific (e.g. Tuesday morning, Saturday afternoon) as this will give the memory a context. This will help you to remember it later.

At first glance it may seem that difficulties remembering what you have just read or where you have parked the car can't be due to a failure to pay attention in the first place. After all, both reading and driving require some concentration. When we first learn to read or drive it takes all of our concentration to complete a task. But as we get older and more experienced these skills, which once took every ounce of concentration, gradually become more and more automatic. In the case of reading, this ability becomes so automatic we just can't inhibit it.

The Stroop Test

There is a famous psychology test based on this principle called the Stroop Test. In the test the subject is presented with a list of colour words like 'blue', 'red', 'yellow', etc. The words are written in different coloured inks and the subject is asked to read the list of words. For anyone who can read, it is a really easy task. But in the second part of the test the subject is asked to ignore the word and tell the experimenter what colour ink the word is written in instead. This is a much, much harder task because our automatic response when we see the word 'yellow' is to read it. To do well on this task the subject has to inhibit the natural response 'yellow' to the word and look at the colour instead. It takes a good deal of concentration not to make a mistake. If you think it sounds easy, you can have a go yourself. (See 'Useful addresses and resources' at the back of this book for 'Stroop Test', page 116.) The test is now so famous it has even been printed on mugs and tee shirts and has been made into a neon art work in a New York gallery.

Once a complex activity becomes automatic, it frees up our brains to do other things at the same time. Thus it is possible to run your eyes over the words on a page but be thinking about something entirely different the whole time. In this situation, reading has become automatic and the meaning of the words just isn't processed deeply enough to allow you to recall it when you turn the page. If you remain distracted, by external things in your environment or your own internal thoughts (or a combination of both), you can read the same page over and over again without much going in at all.

The same 'automatic' principle applies to losing a car in a car park. This tends to happen most frequently in car parks that people are familiar with and have used many times before. Generally when you arrive in a car park you are thinking about where you are going and what you are about to do. You may be late and agitated, or excited, or simply thinking about what you need to buy and, most importantly, what you mustn't forget. Parking the car becomes the secondary task, requiring relatively little brain power as you become focused on what you are about to do. In this situation, it's not particularly surprising that, when you need to find it again, you may find it difficult to remember where exactly you left the car. It's rare that people can't remember which car park they have left their car in; rather, the exact location of the car just wasn't processed properly. In this example, interference from previous memories can also get in the way, and you may automatically return to the bay where you usually park the car, or where you parked it last time. It's also the case that in multi-storey car parks there is often very little to distinguish one floor from another, and what distinguishing features there are (the other cars) are transient and mobile and can't be relied on to trigger any recollections to help you retrace your steps when you return.

These common examples demonstrate that we have to pay attention and process something consciously if we are ever to have a good chance of remembering it later on. While it may sound obvious, it is this failure to pay proper attention to the things we need to remember that underlies many of the most common memory complaints we experience every day. There are many physical and psychological factors that can interfere with how well we manage this on a day-to-day basis. These factors can both enhance and impede our ability to pay proper attention to new information.

The ability to take in new information is the first part of the memory process. Psychologists call this process 'encoding'. It's something you are born with and there can be very wide variations in the normal, healthy population. It's not necessarily related to intelligence. Some people are blessed with an ability to read or hear something once and remember it almost verbatim. Exam revision for these lucky people is a breeze; most of us have to work much harder with active study techniques to cram the information into our brains. Others never forget a face. Very rarely, some people appear to be born with a 'photographic' memory, where they can not only remember things that they have read or seen for a brief period of time, but can also reproduce them, either by drawing or by apparently 'reading' an entire page from memory. However, these people are the exception rather than rule, and as Stephen's story shows, often a phenomenal ability to encode new information appears to develop at the expense of other necessary life skills.

An artist's tale

Stephen Wiltshire was born in London in 1974. He was diagnosed with autism at the age of three and did not learn to speak until the age of nine. Although he had no language and found it difficult to relate to other people he had an incredible talent for drawing and was able to produce detailed and accurate representations of complex cityscapes, often after observing for just a few minutes. He became famous when he demonstrated this unique skill in a BBC documentary where he produced a very detailed and accurate drawing of the Houses of Parliament, entirely from memory. Now an adult, Stephen has continued his career as an artist. He has his own gallery in London and was awarded an MBE for services to the art world in 2006. Despite Stephen's phenomenal memory for architectural detail, his other memory functions aren't out of the ordinary at all. On a visit to New York, he got lost and walked for 45 minutes in the wrong direction before finding his destination.

Some people find that they tend to be better at remembering things that they have read or heard than visual details. Psychologists call this 'verbal' information because it is generally conveyed in words. Other people find that they are better at remembering things visually. Faces are a classic example. Apart from describing a few distinguishing physical features, such as hair colour, a beard or glasses, it is almost impossible to describe someone's face to someone else who hasn't met that person before. Try it now. Think of an acquaintance that you know and try to describe his or her face out loud. It's very difficult and unlikely that anyone listening would get a clear picture of the person you are imagining. Although technology has helped to improve things a little in recent years, our difficulties in translating complex visual images into words are the reason why the police 'photofits' of suspected criminals still tend to look more like characters from the *Beano* than any real-life miscreants.

Bolivian bandits

Bolivian police released this unlikely drawing of a suspect in a murder case in 2009. Incredibly, the release of this picture led to the arrest of the suspect (who turned out to have ears after all!).

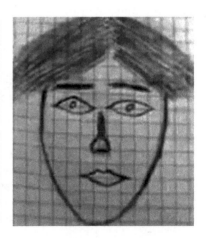

Whether you are better at taking in verbal or visual information, you will have a baseline level at which your memory generally works. You will know from your experiences at school whether you needed to read and re-read (and re-read) your textbooks to get the information to go in, or whether you just seemed to be able to remember what the teacher had said when it came to the exams. You'll know if you have always had a tendency to get lost in a town (or even a building!) or whether you seem to be able to create your own map in your head as you walk around a new place, even to the point of being able to predict where shortcuts might lie. You will know if a new hairstyle on a friend throws you into momentary confusion, or whether you can still recognize a face from your primary school when you see it 20 years later.

How to maximize your encoding

A number of active study techniques have been developed to help maximize the information you take in when you are studying. If you are listening to a talk or a lecture, there is no substitution for taking handwritten notes. Writing notes makes you pay attention and also ensures that information is processed more deeply than it is during passive listening. Unless a lecturer is really engaging, if you just sit and listen you will inevitably drift off during parts of the presentation and may miss a critical piece of information. The only exception to this rule of thumb is in an interactive teaching session that involves a great deal of student participation. In these situations, trying to write everything down can interfere with active participation, which itself is an active study technique. There are a number of guides published on the internet that teach you how to take effective notes in lectures. See the 'Useful addresses and resources' section at the back of this book for more information. Lecture notes do not need to be legible to anyone but yourself. Using abbreviations can increase the amount of information you can take down. If u cn rd ths u cn lrn hw to wrt qckly! To commit the new information to memory you should rewrite your notes as soon as possible after the lecture has finished. Although people are often tempted to type them up on a computer, studies have shown that people remember more when they rewrite notes by hand – again, the information is processed more deeply. If your visual memory is a strength, then you can use visual sketches and annotations and rearrange the information spatially on the page to help you commit it to memory. This re-drafting should always take place in a quiet, calm environment. Even background music or having the radio on can be a distraction. Anything that ensures that the task engages more of your attention will make it more likely that it will stick in your memory. If you rewrite your notes in close proximity to the lecture, you may be able to fill in any gaps from your memory and will also be able to identify anything that doesn't make sense and that you need to clarify.

When it comes to revising for an exam, passive reading is as effective as passive listening is in a lecture – that is, not very! One study with university students found that just sitting and reading a textbook had very little benefit when it came to how well they performed in the subsequent exam. For some, it was actually counterproductive as it gave them an 'illusion of competence'. The students reasoned that since they had spent a while reading the textbook, something must have gone in.

There are a number of acronyms that describe active study techniques to help commit written information to memory; these include the RRR (read, write, review) method, the PQRST (preview, question, read, self-recite, test) method and the SQ3R method (survey, question, read, recite, review). See 'Useful addresses and resources' on page 110 for more information on all of these techniques. All of these approaches encourage maximum processing of information to ensure that it becomes firmly embedded in your memory. All also involve a 'testing' element at the end to make sure that the information has actually gone in. If you have a particularly poor memory (due to illness or underlying brain damage) you may need to repeat these cycles more often than your peers before the information becomes firmly lodged and easily accessible, but the same principles apply to everyone when it comes to committing new information to memory. Chapter 6 describes some of the ways in which you can ease the recall of this information, once it has been committed to memory.

Whatever your baseline ability to take in new information, it can be influenced by a number of different factors that can either enhance or, more often, impede your encoding ability. These changes may be temporary or permanent. Most people begin to notice memory problems when there is a deterioration in their normal level of encoding for one reason or another. The second part of this book describes some of these influences and ways in which you can manipulate some of them to your advantage. Before we move on to this, it's important to understand what happens to information once we have encoded it. The next chapter describes what happens to our 'memories' once they have been properly encoded and redresses some of the most common memory myths that people tend to subscribe to today.

3

Memory myths

Before we go any further, try this test.

Once information has been processed deeply enough to be remembered later, it's tempting to think that that's the end of the story. Many people are familiar with the kind of 'memory' that a computer uses. In computing, the term 'memory' refers to the physical devices that store programs and data. Each stored piece of information is filed away methodically in the computer and can be called up, intact and unchanged, over and over again (notwithstanding an infection with a computer virus).

Unfortunately our brains don't work like that. Although it may not feel like it, your memories of the past are constantly changing and being modified by your later experiences. Pat's story typifies one of the most common complaints that psychologists hear in their memory clinics.

Pat's story

Pat was a 55-year-old social worker who was really worried about how scatty she was becoming at work. She had missed the deadline to deliver critical information on an important case and this had had knock-on effects for her client and the whole team involved in his care. 'I just don't understand it,' she said. 'I can remember my childhood as if it were yesterday, but ask me what I did last week and it's a real struggle to remember.'

Many people who are really troubled by memory problems in their everyday activities are perplexed by the fact that their memory for events in the distant past appears to be crystal clear, like looking through an open window onto the scene. They can often recount, in exquisite detail, numerous events from their childhood. However, these childhood 'memories' have almost always been rehearsed and revisited hundreds of times over the course of a lifetime, whereas what you ate for lunch last Tuesday probably hasn't occupied much of your time or attention since you ate it. So, while someone may have an apparently clear childhood memory of, for example, breaking a window with a cricket ball or falling out of a tree in the woods, that person is very unlikely to be able to give a detailed account of what life was like on an ordinary day at this age. We tend to remember the big events from our childhood: the birth of a sibling, traumatic accidents, seeing something out of the ordinary for the first time. Even with these special events we can usually only recall some key features later on.

The reminiscence bump
Over-rehearsal may not be the only reason that memories from late childhood are so accessible and appear so vivid. Researchers have coined the term 'reminiscence bump' to describe memories from adolescence and early adulthood because individuals typically recall a disproportionate number of memories from this time compared to the rest of their lives. These vivid and varied memories are normally encoded between the ages of 10 and 30. Researchers have come up with a number of explanations for this peak in recall. Some have argued that a great deal of change is usually going on at this time and people tend to remember new and distinct events. Others have argued that this is a period when we fully develop a sense of our own identity and that these memories form part of our personal story of how we became who we are. Whatever the reason, you are by no means unique in having apparent excellent recall of your school days, regardless of the difficulties you may have in finding your car keys every morning.

As we rehearse and revisit these events in our minds and in conversation, these key features form well-worn anecdotes. After a few years, it is these well-rehearsed anecdotes that we remember; very little of the original memory may remain. Since we rarely tell a story without a purpose, every time we tell and retell a story we edit it slightly for the target audience, removing irrelevant material and adding further explanations where necessary. Each time, this editing and retelling adds a subtle layer of distortion, which affects the underlying memory of the event. Although there is sometimes an element of conscious exaggeration for dramatic effect, the typical distortions are largely unconscious and become indistinguishable from the original memory for the storyteller, who absolutely believes his or her recall to be clear and true at each retelling. It's a bit like playing Chinese Whispers with yourself.

Chinese Whispers

Chinese Whispers is a popular children's game played around the world. Players generally sit in a circle or stand in a line and a message or phrase is whispered once from one player to another until the last player announces the message to the whole group. The message has often been significantly distorted by the time the last player hears it, as errors accumulate from one player to the next. The resulting denials and recriminations back down the line can be lively! Chinese Whispers is often used as a metaphor for how rumours spread around a society. Most people wouldn't think that a similar process can happen with their own memories, but it can and has almost certainly happened with some of your most treasured memories of the past.

While it is relatively easy to accept that this distortion may occur over many years, it actually happens far more quickly than you might think. In a series of memory experiments in the 1970s, psychologists in America demonstrated how easy it was to intro-duce false facts into people's memory of events. In one study, the subjects were shown a photograph of two cars that had collided. Half of the subjects were subsequently asked how fast they thought the cars were travelling when they 'hit' each other. The other half were asked how fast the cars were travelling when the cars 'smashed' into each other. Not only did the 'smash' group estimate that the cars were travelling much faster, they were also more likely to 'remember' seeing broken glass from a smashed car window in the picture. There was no broken glass in the original picture. The experimenters went on to ask the subjects about the 'Give Way' sign in the picture. Although they had actually seen a Stop sign in the picture, a number of the subjects also 'remembered' seeing a Give Way sign. The introduction of false cues and leading questions altered participants' memories even though they had only just seen the picture.

Interestingly, once a false memory has been inserted into the original memory it seems to stick there. Subsequent studies have shown that people are more confident in the accuracy of these inserted false details than they are of the real details they witnessed.

This is partly due to the fact that they have been apparently verified and confirmed by a third party. But it may also be due to the pre-existing ideas that people bring to new situations.

There is far too much detail in everyday life for us to remember it all – we just don't have the capacity. To cope with this complexity, we develop simplified, generalized representations of things based on our experience. These representations form from a very young age. Psychologists call these simplified representations 'schemas'. Schemas effectively allow us to summarize events. They are really useful because they don't take up much memory capacity, but they have a downside. We often mistakenly 'recall' events that never really happened, because we associate then with the schema we have developed for that particular event. This distortion has really important implications for the validity of eye-witness testimonies in court cases. Take, for example, a street robbery.

A street robbery
It's raining and Karen has just parked her car outside the bank. She looks across to the cashpoint through the car window and sees an elderly woman at the keypad and a person in jeans and a dark hooded top waiting in line behind her. She realizes that she will need to wait in the small queue to withdraw her cash and so reaches behind her, to the back seat of the car, to retrieve her umbrella. As she opens the car door to get out, she hears a cry and sees the hooded figure running off down the street and the elderly woman crumpled on the floor next to the cashpoint. Karen soon becomes the key witness to the crime and is interviewed by the police.

Witnesses to a crime will inevitably tailor their account (and therefore their memory) to the interests of the listener. The first person that Karen recounts this story to will be critical in shaping and consolidating her memory of the event. If she speaks to other witnesses, their recollections may be incorporated into her memory of the event. This very often happens in real-life witness testimonies where people honestly report seeing things that they couldn't possibly have seen from their viewpoint or position at the scene. In one study, subjects were shown very slightly different versions of a crime filmed from different angles. They were then allowed to talk to each other about what they had seen. A statement was then taken as if they were talking to the police. An incredible 70 per cent of the subjects reported at least one thing in their statements that they could not possibly have seen themselves.

In taking her witness statement, the police may ask Karen how old she thought the boy was. Immediately the suspected criminal has been identified as a male in Karen's mind. In actual fact, she only saw the back of a hooded figure in androgynous clothes. This false memory may have been inserted by the leading question, but will also have been helped along by Karen's pre-existing ideas about street crime. Karen's general schema for robberies at cashpoints probably already involves young men in hoodies. This schema is then reinforced by the police questions.

In addition to shaping our memories of events, schemas also often fill in gaps in our recollections. By the end of the day, Karen may be 100 per cent certain that she witnessed a robbery earlier in the day, when in fact she actually only saw the scene before and after the event. When there are small gaps in what we see, we tend to fill in the gaps with pre-existing schema for the event.

Mind the gap

On the morning of Thursday 7 July 2005, four suicide bombers detonated bombs on three tube trains and a bus in London. Over 50 people were killed in the attacks, and more than 700 were injured. Two weeks later, four more terrorists attempted to replicate the attack. They failed, but escaped and were still at large on the following day. Consequently the entire population of London was on high alert for terrorists. The day after the failed attack, Mr Jean Charles de Menezes walked through the barrier at Stockwell tube station using his Oyster card to pay his fare and picked up a free newspaper on the way. He was wearing a light denim jacket and descended the escalator. He ran across the platform as his train arrived and took his seat on the train. Having been falsely identified as one of the fugitive failed bombers from the previous day, Mr de Menezes was then shot by members of the anti-terrorist squad and died at the scene. On the day Mr de Menezes was killed, a picture rapidly emerged from multiple eye witnesses who reported seeing him vaulting over the ticket barrier and running away from the police down into the tube station. Witnesses said he was wearing a heavy winter coat on the warm summer's day, raising suspicions that it was concealing a device. One witness even reported seeing Mr de Menezes wearing a bomb belt with wires sticking out. None of these things were true, but all fitted the vivid collective schema of how a terrorist might look and behave.

The Jean Charles de Menezes case is a good example of how people both consciously and unconsciously tailor their accounts of events to the interests of the listener. The majority of the initial eye-witness accounts in this case were given to reporters who are trained to elicit dramatic accounts from their sources and who were competing for the best eye witness to put in front of their cameras. Leading questions and inaccurate corroborative accounts from other witnesses served to create a spiral of false recollections, based on the incorrect presumption that a terrorist had been caught.

When they are talking to the police, eye witnesses tend to remember more incriminating details than neutral or exonerating facts. It's an unconscious bias based on the knowledge that the police are looking to catch the criminal. In Karen's story, for example, she is unlikely to tell the police that rain was partly obscuring the view through her car window, or that she reached into the back seat of the car for her umbrella and did not have her eyes on the scene when the robbery actually took place. Exonerating details can soon be forgotten or dismissed as the story is repeated. In TV courtroom dramas and real-life court cases, barristers can often belittle any details that an eye witness may suddenly remember on the witness stand if they were not included in the original witness statement, particularly if they cast doubt on the guilt of a suspect. This is despite that fact that scientific studies of the way in which memory works suggest that any fresh recollection of details at this stage may be more accurate than the incriminating details, which will have been well rehearsed.

These psychology studies and real-life examples emphasize just how unreliable our memories are. Even when the brain is working properly and we have full confidence in our recollections, we will have seen what we wanted or expected to see and will have then organized the information in a way that made sense. Fortunately there are some effective techniques that can be used to try to counter some of these natural biases and distortions to improve the accuracy of our recall.

Studies have shown that people's memory improves if they physically revisit the scene of an event. Features in the environment can trigger new recollections. The sooner someone gives an account of an event after it has happened, the more detail he or she is likely to remember later. The police interview technique that elicits the most information from eye witnesses to a crime is called the cognitive interview. Rather than just asking for a chronological account of events, the technique uses four strategies designed to maximize recall. These are:

1 Mentally recreating the environmental and personal context that existed at the time of the event. This involves both visualizing the scene and thinking about your frame of mind at the time. Where had you just been? What had just happened? What were you expecting to do next?
2 Recording everything regardless of its perceived importance. Try to remember every detail, even if it doesn't seem relevant to the main event – each detail may trigger a new recollection that is important.
3 Recounting events in a variety of different orders can often bring to light new information.
4 Similarly, recalling the events from a variety of perspectives can also bring out new details.

Remember the word list at the beginning of the chapter? Before you read on, take a moment now to write down in a notepad as many of the words as you can remember.

About half of the people who do this test will remember 'window' as one of the words. It wasn't in the original list, but most of the words had a connection to 'window': curtain, glass, glaze, frame, etc. In addition you have read the word 'window' no fewer than five times in this chapter since you looked at the list.

Page 20: Many people who are really troubled by memory problems in their everyday activities are perplexed by the fact that their memory for events in the distant past appears to be crystal clear, like looking through an open *window* onto the scene.

Page 20: So while someone may have an apparently clear childhood memory of, for example, breaking a *window* with a cricket ball or falling out of a tree in the woods, that person is very unlikely to be able to give a detailed account of what life was like on an ordinary day at this age.

Page 22: Not only did the 'smash' group estimate that the cars were travelling much faster, they were also more likely to 'remember' seeing broken glass from a smashed car *window* in the picture.

Page 23: She looks across to the cashpoint through the car *window* and sees an elderly woman at the keypad and a person in jeans and a dark hooded top waiting in line behind her.

Page 25: In Karen's story, for example, she is unlikely to tell the police that rain was partly obscuring the view through her car *window* . . .

If you incorrectly remembered that the word 'window' was in the original list at the beginning of this chapter, you are not alone and have just demonstrated to yourself how easily memory can be distorted. If not, don't congratulate yourself too much; these processes will be at work in your brain too and will catch you out sooner or later.

Summary

On the whole we tend to trust our memories, yet it is not necessary for us to lie or be deliberately economical with the truth to inaccurately state the facts in any situation. Just being human is enough to create distorted recall and inaccurate recollections on a daily basis.

Memory does not work like a video recording of past events. The very act of laying down each new memory creates distortions which in turn will interfere with both the subsequent recollections of previous events and the laying down of future memories. Much of what we recall from the past is not an accurate representation of what actually happened. The way we organize information and impose meaning on it creates our own, somewhat fluid, version of events. While the key facts may be accurate, many of the details will be subject to interference from a wide variety of sources. This is artfully expressed by the novelist Marcelo Figueras in his novel *Kamchatka*.

> Sometimes there are variations in what I remember . . . these variations don't worry me. I'm used to them. They mean I'm remembering something I hadn't noticed before; they mean that I am not exactly the same person I was when I last remembered.

The next time you are perplexed that you can remember your school days as if they were yesterday but not what you did last week, take heart from the realization that you are not reaching back over decades, but actually only back to the last time you re-rehearsed either a special memory or a deeply entrenched routine from that time. These 'memories' just aren't comparable to the humdrum things you did last week, which you probably haven't given a second thought since. There is no mystery in the apparent paradox at all.

4

You never forget how to ride a bike

The previous chapters have explained how many everyday memory complaints are due to the fact that information hasn't been processed properly in the first place and how, even when we do pay attention, our most precious memories can be subject to all kinds of bias and distortions from the very first time we recall them. Everything that has been discussed so far has been in the context of remembering things that have happened in the past. Psychologists call this kind of memory 'episodic memory' – the memory for episodes. We can also think of it as autobiographical memory – the memory of things that have happened to us. While these kinds of memories make up the bulk of our personal recollections there are a number of other memory systems in our brains that appear to work in a different way and that don't seem to be subject to the same distortions.

Procedural memories

The knowledge of 'how' to do something is stored in the brain in a very different way from our memories of past events. People often say, 'You never forget how to ride a bike', and it's generally true. Once you have mastered a skill, it tends to stay with you. You may not have ridden a bike for 30 years, but notwithstanding a few nervous wobbles to begin with, you will be able to ride a bike within minutes, if you were proficient as a child. It just comes back to you, without you needing to think about it consciously at all. Psychologists call this 'procedural memory' – the memory needed to perform particular types of action or procedure. Procedural memories are processed in our subconscious; once a skill is learnt, it doesn't require any effortful thinking to retrieve it and put it into action. Our bodies/brains just seem to know what to do. Whenever they are needed, procedural memories are automatically retrieved.

From getting dressed to reading the paper, playing a musical instrument to driving a car, once we have mastered these skills, we tend not to forget them.

Although procedural memories are easily retrieved once they have been created, it is by no means easy to get a skill into procedural memory. Procedural memories are created through 'procedural learning' – the repetition of an action over and over again until it becomes automatic. The more complicated the skill, the more difficult it is to commit to procedural memory. Fortunately we do most of our procedural learning when we are children. The young brain is primed to make all the connections it needs to acquire new skills. Few of us can remember the effort it takes to 'sound out' words phonetically in order to read them, but time spent with any young child learning to read illustrates the effort required to master the skill before it becomes automatic. New skills always demand 100 per cent attention and concentration from the learner at the outset. It is often difficult to imagine that they will ever require anything less when you start to acquire a new skill. You may remember this feeling after a first driving lesson. But with more and more practice, more and more aspects of the skill become automatic until eventually the entire procedure is committed to procedural memory.

Sometimes a procedure or skill becomes so automatic that it's difficult to even remember doing it at all. The action becomes so automatic and unconscious, we do not process it sufficiently to enable us to recall it later. Most of us have experienced the momentary disconcertion where you go to do something, like locking the back door before you go out, only to find that you have already done it. The action was so automatic, you just didn't process it the first time. The fact that you encounter the unexpected (an already locked door) when you go to do it again jolts the action to consciousness. Similarly, experienced drivers may be familiar with the sudden realization that they have not been aware of a recent chunk of their journey. This realization is often triggered by an unexpected event which suddenly forces an aspect of driving into conscious control. Prior to that, they have been driving 'automatically', freeing up their conscious mind to think about other things. This phenomenon is not limited to mundane daily activities.

Expertise-induced amnesia

In the 2010 Winter Olympics, arch rivals Canada and the USA reached the ice hockey final. The game was closely fought, and with the two teams evenly matched it went to overtime. In the dying seconds of the game a Canadian player, Sidney Crosby, clinched the match with an audacious goal, securing the Olympic gold medal for his country. The moment will be etched into the minds of millions of ice hockey fans. Experts later determined that Crosby had made over 20 decisions in the four-second crucible of action in which he initiated and finished the goal sequence. But when he was interviewed immediately after the match Crosby had no real memory of the events. When he was asked by a reporter to talk through the goal he replied, 'I don't really remember, I just shot it – I think from around here . . . that's all I really remember . . . um, I didn't really see it, to be honest.'

Interestingly, studies that have used MRI scans to look at brain activity suggest that people with Obsessive Compulsive Disorder (OCD) perform considerably better on procedural memory tasks than people without the disorder. These studies suggest that procedural memory in OCD patients is unusually good, particularly in the early learning stages of acquiring a new skill. This may mean that people with OCD develop 'expertise amnesia' more quickly and for a wider range of actions than people without the disorder, creating the initial trigger for 'checking' that tasks have been done, as they cannot recall doing them. Treatment approaches based on these ideas involve deliberately bringing some aspects of the automatic, over-learned behaviour back into conscious control. As discussed in Chapter 2, the most simple way to do this is to say something out loud as you complete the action, such as 'I am locking the back door' or 'I have turned off the light.' For more complicated actions that require several steps (e.g. packing to go on holiday), conscious confirmation that an action has been completed can be achieved using pencil and paper checklists or specialist apps on mobile phones.

Psychological choking

Procedural memories are generally very robust and resistant, but they can be disrupted by very high levels of stress. This is often happens when someone is required to perform the skill in front of other people. It is as if access to the procedural memory store is suddenly blocked and the person performs like a beginner again. This is often seen in the sporting arena, where sportspeople appear to crumble as the pressure builds and often end up just 'giving' the game to their opponents, to the incredulity of their fans. This phenomenon is often referred to as 'choking' and there are some infamous examples in the sporting world. Greg Norman's performance in the 1996 Golf Masters Tournament frequently tops the polls of the worst sporting collapses. Entering the final round, Norman had a six-stroke lead over Nick Faldo. That's a big lead in golf, but not big enough if you start to choke. By the 11th hole Faldo had closed the gap. At the very next hole, Norman dropped two shots. His game fell apart and he eventually finished five shots behind Faldo.

Psychologists think this happens because stress increases the performers' self-consciousness. In other words, they start to think about what they are doing. This focus overrides access to their well-learned, automatic skills. What was effortless and unconscious when the game began becomes slow and deliberate as the pressure builds. A vicious circle is quickly established. This is why the performance of some sportspeople appears to collapse so quickly and so spectacularly in the final stages of a game.

The England football team and the curse of the penalty shootout

Penalty shootouts are a nerve-racking way to settle a football match. They were introduced to the World Cup in 1982, when replays were no longer practicable given the disruption they caused to players, fans and (primarily) the worldwide television schedules. England faced their first penalty shootout in 1990, in the World Cup semi-final, after drawing 1–1 with West Germany. A huge amount was riding on the outcome of the shootout: not just a chance to defeat arch rivals Germany, but a place for England in their first World Cup final since 1966. All went well until the German goalkeeper saved Stuart Pearce's goal. At 3–4 to Germany, Chris Waddle *had* to score to keep England in the tournament. Incredibly, his shot missed the goal completely and sailed over the crossbar. Disbelieving schoolchildren and pundits alike couldn't comprehend how a world-class football player could miss the goal entirely.

Critics say the penalty shootout is little better than a coin toss when it comes to determining which is the better team. It may not be the best test of footballing skill but it does seem to be a good test of the ability to stay calm under pressure, and not choke. If it were down to chance, one would predict a fairly even spread of wins and losses across the teams. This is not the case. Since its introduction, the England football team have played eight matches in major tournaments which have gone to a penalty kick shootout. They have only won one, while Germany have yet to lose a penalty shootout in a World Cup tournament.

Choking is not limited to the sporting arena; concert pianists, public speakers and even mere mortals like us can all experience 'choking' when the pressure is such that we temporarily lose access to our procedural memory store. A world championship doesn't need to be at stake to induce 'choking'; sometimes it may just be the threat of a parking ticket.

Annie's story

Annie came to our memory clinic very concerned about an upsetting incident that had occurred in the supermarket the previous week. 'It was just awful,' she said. 'I was staring into my purse and just couldn't work out which coins to give the cashier. My mind went blank . . . the more I looked, the more scared I got. I could see that the cashier was getting impatient and the man behind me in the queue was sighing and huffing and puffing. In the end I just handed my purse over to her to get the money out herself. I felt such a fool. I haven't been back to the shop since.'

When we talked to Annie a little more about this incident, it transpired that on the day this had happened she had parked on a double yellow line outside the supermarket and was keen to get back to her car as soon as possible to avoid a parking ticket. In her haste, she had inadvertently joined an 'eight items or less' queue with her basket of goods. Although she only had a small basket, it contained more than eight items. She had apologized to the cashier but had not received a reassuring response, although her apology did elicit a 'hurrumph' from the man behind her in the queue. It is likely that Annie's anxiety about getting a parking ticket and her embarrassment about being in the wrong queue induced a sufficient amount of stress for her to temporarily lose access to her procedural memory, blocking her ability to complete the simple transaction at the till. We discussed this possibility with Annie, and spent a few sessions working on ways to help her recognize when her stress levels were high and the role that her anxiety about memory problems might be contributing to this stress. She also received some training in stress management techniques. At her follow-up appointment 12 months later, she was visibly more relaxed than when we first met her and her problems with money had not recurred.

Summary

Procedural memories (memories for how to do something) can be very hard to acquire. They generally take a lot of practice and repetition to create. Many of our procedural memories are created in childhood when the brain is primed, ready to make all the connections it needs to master new skills. Generally speaking, the older you are the harder it is to commit a new skill to procedural memory. That doesn't mean it's impossible to learn a new language or to play an new instrument as an adult, just that it will take more repetition and practice than for someone with a younger brain. Once a skill has been committed to procedural memory and we have mastered it to the point that it becomes automatic and subconscious, procedural memories are very resistant to deterioration. This can be a mixed blessing. When we are functioning on 'automatic' it frees up brain capacity for other things, but this means that we may not always process actions and events properly. Sometimes it can be helpful to bring back some aspects of the behaviour into conscious control, to ensure that we can remember it later on. The easiest way to do this is to create a commentary for yourself. Procedural memories can be disrupted when someone is under pressure and feeling stressed. In the absence of high levels of stress, regular and/ or progressive difficulties in accessing procedural memories may be a sign of neurological disease. See Chapter 9 for more information.

5
Remembering to remember

In the topsy-turvy world of *Alice in Wonderland*, Alice is thrown into confusion when she meets the White Queen in the woods. Just after the Queen has explained the 'jam' rule (for the uninitiated, it's 'jam tomorrow and jam yesterday – but never jam today') she goes on to explain how memory works both ways. 'I'm sure mine only works one way,' Alice replies. 'I can't remember things before they happen.' The Queen retorts that 'It's a poor sort of memory that only works backwards.'

Although this exchange is supposed to illustrate the non-sensical Wonderland world of the White Queen, Lewis Carroll inadvertently touches on a truism in these words. We do rely on our memories reaching into the future when we need to remember to do something. Psychologists call this 'prospective memory' – remembering to remember. Prospective memory has three components. The first is an intention to do something later: for example, 'I must post Sam's birthday card.' The second key feature is a delay between forming the intention and actually carrying it out. This delay is typically filled with activities that are unrelated to the intention. The third feature is the absence of an explicit prompt indicating that it is time to carry out the action (like an alarm) – you just need to remember to remember, at the right time, in the right place.

Psychologists have estimated that at least half of our forgetting is due to the failure of prospective memory. This isn't really surprising when you think about it. Regardless of employment status, our days are generally spent forming intentions and then acting on them. It's not surprising, then, that some of these intentions never get fulfilled. Prospective memories can relate to set daily routines, such as taking medications at regular times, or to irregular one-offs, such as posting a letter or remembering to attend a medical appointment or to pick up a pint of milk on your way home.

Failures of prospective memory can cause more than just irritation and inconvenience. Every day in the UK, one in ten patients fails to attend his or her NHS appointment. This costs the country millions of pounds. Some of the people who fail to turn up have legitimate reasons for their 'no show'; after all, illness and death are common among hospital patients. Poor communication between the hospital and the patients has also been blamed for a sizable proportion of the 'no shows', with hospital letters frequently going astray or sent to the wrong patient entirely. However, it is estimated that a startling 50 per cent of all missed appointments may be due to the patient simply forgetting all about it.

A recent study suggested that the number of patients failing to turn up for hospital appointments could be reduced by a third by using text messages or phone reminders. However, the patients who took part in the study didn't just need a simple memory jog. Interestingly, the researchers found that automated reminders (like texts and emails) were less effective than the hospital staff telephoning the patients before the appointment and speaking to them personally. The personal reminders produced a 39 per cent reduction in 'no shows' while the figure was only 29 per cent for automated reminders. It seems that there is something about the personal interaction that 'bumps' the appointment up the patient's priority list when it comes to prospective memory. This may be because, once you have been telephoned and a personal dimension has been added into the equation, engendering the possible sense of letting someone else down, the consequences of not attending the appointment have become greater.

Different countries tackle this problem in different ways. In Canada, patients are fined about £30 if they fail to attend their appointments, while in Germany it is considered extremely bad manners not to show up, generating a social stigma. Whatever the mechanism, it seems that the prospective memory failures that afflict so many when it comes to appointments can be reduced if the probable consequences of the failure are increased. Although this principle has been used to try to change the behaviour of large groups of people, it can also be used to reduce prospective memory failures in individuals. Strategies based on these principles that you can use in everyday life are discussed at the end of this chapter.

Millions of people must remember to take medications every day to maintain their health. The consequences of not taking medication regularly are different for different conditions, but in many instances the consequences of forgetting the odd dose may not be immediately felt. A recent Australian study interviewed over 4,000 elderly people with high blood pressure about their medication and how often they took it. Unsurprisingly, they found that people who took all their medications regularly, and at the specified time, were less likely to have a heart attack and die than those who didn't take their medication as prescribed. However, they also found that people who answered 'yes' to the question 'Do you ever forget to take your medication?' were significantly more likely to experience a heart attack than those who answered 'no'. The striking thing about this study is that it didn't look at how often people forgot to take their blood pressure medications, just whether they ever forgot.

Your life in their hands

Sometimes the consequences of prospective memory failures can be catastrophic. Airline pilots must remember to perform several actions prior to taking off, to ensure the safety of the plane and its passengers. These actions are usually performed in a set routine to ensure that none of the steps are missed. Yet a team at NASA found that the inadvertent omission of an entirely routine procedural step by the crew played a pivotal role in five of the 27 major US airline accidents that occurred between 1987 and 2001. In each of these accidents, a highly experienced pilot had forgotten to perform a crucial procedural step, one that he or she had always performed, without difficulty or error, on thousands of previous flights.

The NASA team were determined to find out why these normal routine steps had been bypassed by the crew. They found that all the pilots had been interrupted when they were performing cockpit procedures, especially when they were at the departure gate. Cabin crew, gate crew, mechanics and air traffic controllers frequently break into the long sequence of checks that pilots need to complete before they start the engines. The most common error the pilots made after these interruptions was to go on to the next task in the routine, rather than to go back to what they were doing at the time and ensure that it was complete. As a result of these studies, cockpit procedures were changed and external reminders (lights and beeps) were introduced to alert the pilots to the fact that the task was not complete. Instructing pilots about the effect of interruptions, and using psychological strategies to make them consciously aware that the task had been interrupted, was also effective in reducing these errors.

Ageing and prospective memory

Although wisdom may increase as we get older, there is no getting away from the fact that there are many aspects of cognitive function that deteriorate (see Chapter 12). When it comes to prospective memory, the research is mixed regarding the effect of ageing. Some studies have found that older people are far more prone to prospective memory failures than younger people, while others have found no differences at all. Some psychologists think that age-related declines in prospective memory are even larger than the age-related declines seen in retrospective memory. Others have argued that prospective memory is an exception to the rule and that it holds up and remains completely intact across the adult lifespan.

In 2008, a scientist from Canada decided to settle the controversy using a meta-analysis. A meta-analysis is a giant review that pulls together all of the data from all of the studies on a particular topic and combines the results. This often identifies the sources of disagreement among the researchers. The meta-analysis on prospective memory and ageing found that prospective memory does decline with ageing. Studies that reported no age-related declines in prospective memory hadn't been designed properly. Sometimes the tests were too easy, so everyone was able to do them regardless of their age. Sometimes the tests weren't really proper tests of prospective memory, because the people were given hints and prompts to carry out their previous intentions. For example, they might be told to ask the experimenter for a cup of tea when they heard a buzzer, rather than at a specific time. The meta-analysis suggested that while there weren't large age differences in the ability to perform prospective memory tasks in response to prompts (like buzzers and alarms, etc.), older people were significantly worse in real-life tasks that didn't provide any prompts or reminders – such as remembering to pick something up from the supermarket on the way home. Fortunately we can use the fact that we do not lose the ability to respond to prompts, cues and memory jogs to help develop effective strategies to overcome the natural age-related decline in the ability to spontaneously become aware of our previous plans at the right time and in the right place.

Strategies for remembering to remember

A number of strategies have been devised to try to reduce the impact of procedural memory failures. Although some were developed in response to very specific problems (such as the forgetfulness of pilots) the principles upon which they are based apply to all of us and they can be adapted to help us with everyday memory problems.

Upping the ante

The more important something is, the less likely we are to forget it. If your daughter is getting married next Saturday, it is unlikely that you will forget to go to the wedding – the consequences of doing so would be huge. The same cannot be said for forgetting to attend a routine eye test scheduled for next Tuesday. One way of increasingly the likelihood that you will remember to remember is to increase the importance of the event, and the consequences if you forget. Take the example of a hospital appointment. If you only envisage a failure to attend as a minor inconvenience to yourself, the consequences of forgetting the appointment will be less than if you consider the wider implications for the doctor who is waiting for you and the patients who could have been seen in your place. By upping the ante and increasing the potential consequences of a memory lapse you can increase the likelihood that you will remember to remember.

Visualization

Visualization can also have a significant effect on remembering to remember. Visualizing an action, together with a clear statement of intent, can make it significantly more likely that you will remember to do something later on. So, if you want to remember to stop off on the way home and buy some milk, you might visualize yourself driving towards the corner shop and pulling up outside. As you are visualizing this you can say out loud, 'When I drive past the pub I will remember to turn left to pick up some milk from the corner shop.' Studies have shown that this joint approach of visualization and explicitly stating intentions out loud is particularly effective at helping older people to remember and act upon their plans.

The impact of interruptions

The studies of pilot errors show just how important interruptions can be in derailing our intentions. Any kind of distraction or interruption can interfere with what we are doing and can lead to mistakes and errors. Just being aware of this can help. Whenever you are interrupted, recognize the fact. Mentally acknowledging, 'I have been interrupted' and asking yourself, 'What was I doing?' and, 'Where had I got to?' can ensure that you return to the correct place in a sequence of actions and can bring your initial intentions back to the forefront of your mind.

Prompts and reminders

Probably the most effective way of reducing the likelihood that you will forget to remember is to make sure that you have plenty of prompts and reminders along the way. Traditional to-do lists are one of the most effective ways of propping up prospective memory. In our digital age, numerous apps for smartphones have also been developed that can be programmed with bleeps or even spoken commands in your own voice, set to go off at specific times to remind you of what you need to do (or should be doing). Although the schedules can be complex to set up, once they are up and running these electronic prompts can be very effective indeed. All prospective memory tasks can be reduced to just one action – remembering to take the phone with you. Some memory prompts are physical. Drug wallets or tablet boxes are plastic boxes divided into individual compartments representing the morning, afternoon and evening of every day of the week. At a set time every week (usually Sunday evenings) you can place all your medication for the week into the correct compartment. It is then easy to check every day whether you have taken your medication or not.

Summary

Prospective memory refers to our ability to become aware of a previously formed plan at the right time and place. The consequences of these memory failures can range from mild irritation to devastating loss of life. Our ability to remember to remember deteriorates with age, but fortunately the performance of older people can be brought into line with that of younger people if prompts are introduced to jog their memory. In our digital age it has never been easier to integrate these reminders into our lives. In the absence of pen and paper and digital bells and whistles, there are a number of psychological strategies you can employ which have been proven to reduce prospective memory problems in everyday life, including upping the ante, visualization and recognizing the impact of interruption on intentions.

6

When it all comes flooding back . . .

The previous chapters have described some of the ways in which you can maximize your chances of committing something to memory. While many memory complaints are actually due to the fact that information was never properly processed in the first place, memory difficulties can also arise when you try to retrieve information from your long-term store and your access seems to be blocked. This information has been properly processed and you often *know* it's there. You may be able to recall all kinds of peripheral details, but the key point you want to remember remains elusive. Some people have likened the experience to looking through a shuttered shop window. You know it's the right shop and can see glimpses of what you want through the gaps and holes in the shutters, but the complete picture remains obscured. Difficulties in recalling information you know you know can be incredibly frustrating. This chapter looks at some of the reasons why these blocks occur when we try to retrieve information from our long-term memory store and discusses some strategies that can aid retrieval.

What causes blocking?

As discussed in the previous chapters, memory is a dynamic process, subject to all kinds of interference. However much it seems to the contrary, memory is not analogous to a video recording of our experience. Everybody has a tendency to forget facts over time, even things that we once knew well. Human memory works rather like a museum. If an exhibit isn't very interesting and it is never looked at, it may be moved to a back room or put into storage where it may fade and begin to decay. Eventually it may be cleared out to make way for more interesting exhibits. Psychologists think that this is what happens to old memories that are very rarely retrieved or revisited. This is beneficial as it makes way for more useful memories. Sometimes we can't retrieve information from our long-term memory store because only fragments remain, or it simply isn't there any more.

Often when we go to retrieve one memory, another similar one comes to mind and 'blocks' access to the thing we really want to recall. This becomes more common as people get older, partly because the memories of a lifetime have similar characteristics and begin to 'overlap'. This can sometimes cause memories to 'merge' together and features from one memory can become incorporated into another. The cues for one memory may be very similar to another: same place, same people, same time of year, etc. In these situations one memory may come to the fore when you are trying to remember something else and this prominent memory will 'block' access to others that are similar. Research has suggested that about half of all 'blocked' memories are correctly retrieved within about a minute of trying to remember. This process is quicker if someone is trying to recall something in a calm, quiet environment. It may not happen for hours (or even days) if you are trying to recall something in a busy, noisy environment and feel under a great deal of pressure.

Improving access

Although we tend to relive our memories verbally, primarily by talking about them, a large amount of sensory information is also encoded and attached to our memories of past events, including smells, tastes and sounds. Exposure to these cues again, even after a long time, can often trigger 'involuntary memories'. Involuntary memories are rich 'snapshots' of past events that suddenly burst into consciousness, apparently from nowhere. Although they may seem completely unconnected to where you are or what you are doing at the time, these memories can be triggered by long-forgotten smells and tastes from the past, or by connections with your present situation that may be subconscious.

Proust's madeleine

The French writer Marcel Proust's encounter with a madeleine cake is the most celebrated literary account of an involuntary memory. Presented with a cup of tea and a madeleine cake as an adult, the writer was suddenly transported back to his childhood, with a vivid recollection of his Sunday morning routine at his aunt's house. In *Remembrance of Things Past* he wrote:

> No sooner had the warm liquid mixed with the crumbs reached my lips than a shudder ran through me and I stopped, fully focused on the extraordinary thing that was happening to me. An exquisite pleasure had invaded my senses, with no suggestion of its origin . . . love was filling me with a precious essence . . . Where did it come from? What did it mean? How could I grasp and understand it? . . . And suddenly the memory revealed itself. The taste was that of the little piece of madeleine which on Sunday mornings at Combray . . . when I went to say good morning to her in her bedroom, my aunt Léonie used to give me, dipping it first in her own cup of tea or tisane. The sight of the little madeleine had recalled nothing to my mind before I tasted it.

Although sensory cues are powerful triggers for involuntary memories, they can also be harnessed to improve access to memories you consciously want to recall. It's easier to retrieve a memory when you are in the same psychological state as you were when the memory was encoded. Being in the same place, smelling the same aromas and tasting the same food will all help to bring back memories. Of course, it is often not possible to physically re-create the scene, but mentally reconstructing as many elements as you can remember will help you to recall. This phenomenon can be used to a student's advantage in exam situations. Revising in the same place that you will take the exam may not be possible, but it might be possible to pair a distinctive perfume or aftershave with the revision and the exam and to chew on the same gum, or suck the same sweets, in both situations. Every little helps when it comes to easing memories from your long-term store.

Sometimes memories are so bound up with the psychological and physiological state the person was in when they were formed that they remain completely inaccessible until that state is reached again. The most common instance is of memories that are created under the influence of alcohol or drugs. People often become amnesic for events when they are drunk. However, if they are in a similar state again, and find themselves in the same place, some memories can 'come back' and appear to be unlocked.

A drinker's tale

In 1835, Dr John Elliotson reported the case of one of his patients who worked in a warehouse. When he was sober, the porter had no memories of what he had done when he was drunk, and vice versa. On one occasion he lost a valuable parcel while he was drunk. When he was sober he had absolutely no recollection of ever seeing the parcel. However, the next time he was intoxicated, he remembered where he had wrongly delivered the parcel and was able to successfully retrieve it. Dr Elliotson concluded that 'the man must have had two souls, one for his sober state, and one for him when drunk'.

Word-finding difficulties

Word-finding difficulties can be one of the most frustrating 'blocks' of all. Word-finding difficulties occur when you *know* what word you want but just can't quite retrieve it. It may be the name of an actor or the title of a film you have seen. Often it's possible to recall all kinds of other details, and people may even know what letter the elusive name begins with, but the actual name remains tantalizingly just out of reach. Word-finding difficulties can sometimes occur with ordinary words in general conversation. As with other memory blocks, the frequency of word-finding difficulties increases with age. The correct word is always immediately recognized if someone else supplies it or when it eventually comes back.

There are a number of strategies that can help with word-finding difficulties. There are two useful kinds of memory jogs that may help to 'release' the elusive name: using clues that relate to the sound of the word and clues that relate to its meaning. Knowing what letter the word begins with and how many syllables it has can help retrieval. Sometimes the beginning sound is available, sometimes it is necessary to mentally run through the alphabet to find the right letter. Another strategy is to try and think of words that might rhyme with the missing word. Clues related to the category or background of the word can also help to unblock it. For example, if you are trying to remember the name of an actor in a particular film, you can try to think about some of the other films he has appeared in and his co-stars. In the same way that taking a run-up to leap over a ditch is more effective than jumping from a standing start, sometimes taking a verbal run-up to find a word can also help to release it. This can be done by constructing a sentence with the elusive word at the end. For example, if you are trying to recall the name of the actress who starred in *Casablanca*, you might say to yourself, '*Casablanca* starred Humphrey Bogart as Rick and the character of Ilsa was played by . . .' Using category clues you might mentally compile a list of items of the same type; in this case it might be famous actresses from the 1940s or other films in which she might have starred.

In casual conversation, other people can often supply the elusive word you are searching for. However, in more formal situations, word-finding difficulties can be embarrassing. If you are worried about word-finding difficulties in a formal presentation it is often useful to write down the key names and phrases you will be using and keep these in sight on a small cue card during your speech. Often just the process of writing these words down beforehand ensures that they remain accessible when you need to use them, and the cue card isn't actually needed. However, if you have it ready, it will also lessen your anxiety and reduce the likelihood of word-finding difficulties occurring. In formal social situations, circumlocution may be the only way around a specific word block. Circumlocution is using many words for something when a concise and commonly used word or expression already exists. Fortunately social conversations contain many circumlocutions – extraneous words fuel fluid conversations – so the occasional wordy explanation may well go unnoticed. Indeed, other people may provide the elusive word without ever realizing that you have temporarily lost access to it. While occasional word-finding difficulties are very common and nothing to worry about, loss of access to the words for common everyday items or word-finding difficulties that significantly interfere with an individual's ability to conduct everyday conversations may be a sign of something more worrying: see Chapter 14.

Summary

The more deeply encoded information is and the more often you retrieve it, the easier it is to recall. It is easier to remember things you have experienced than things you have been told. Putting yourself into the same psychological and physiological state as you were when the memory was encoded will help you to recall it later. Sights, sounds, tastes and smells can all be powerful memory triggers, as can emotional states. Sometimes, though, these cues are common to a number of events, and a specific occasion that you are trying to recall can become blocked by similar memories. Trying to 'force' a memory into consciousness rarely works. However, thinking around the event and asking questions such as 'Was it hot or cold? What were you wearing? What did you eat?' – anything that puts the event in a wider personal context – can help to unlock elusive memories. These sensory cues can also be used to maximize the chances of recall when you know your memory will be tested at a specific time and place in the future, such as in examinations. Word-finding difficulties can be the most frustrating of 'blocks' when it comes to retrieving something from your long-term store that you know is there. Fortunately there are a number of strategies that can lessen the nuisance of these difficulties in everyday life.

Part 2
HOW MEMORY GOES WRONG

7

Anxiety, stress and depression

It's almost impossible to over-emphasize the impact that stress, anxiety and depression can have on your memory function. Between them, these three states are responsible for the overwhelming majority of serious memory problems in otherwise healthy individuals. They also exacerbate memory problems in people with neurological conditions. Regardless of whether your memory complaints are due to an underlying physical condition, medication, hormonal changes or any other cause, gaining control over the levels of stress and anxiety in your life and tackling any underlying depression will have a beneficial impact on your memory function. This chapter explains the ways in which each of these three states interferes with memory function and describes some of the ways that you may be able to lessen the impact.

Stress and memory

Stress is distinct from both anxiety and depression. Stress refers to anything that puts a system under pressure and disturbs its natural equilibrium. In the case of the human body, this stress can take many forms. It may have an external, physical source, such as excessive noise, light or pollution. The human body can also be stressed on a physiological level by poor nutrition, obesity, illness or drugs that are introduced into the system. Probably the most familiar form of stress we encounter on a day-to-day basis is the psychological kind. These forms of stress often merge into each other. Many people find their workplace stressful and feel exhausted after a day's work. Harsh lighting, difficult colleagues and looming deadlines with no time for lunch all mean that the body will have been subjected to a wide range of stressors by the end of the working day. Knowing that it all starts again in a few hours can add to the burden. Very high levels of stress can also be induced by life events over which we have little control, for example illness and death of our loved ones, relationship breakdown and unemployment, not to mention living with a teenager.

The discomfort we feel when we are stressed is part of the human body's response to a perceived threat or danger. As soon as we become aware of a threat, or sometimes just the increased possibility of danger, our body reacts by releasing hormones such as cortisol and adrenaline, getting us ready for action. These chemicals make us more alert and physically prepare our muscles so that we are ready to either fight or run away fast. This is called the flight–fight response.

Far back in our evolutionary history, almost all the threats we faced were probably to life and limb. However, the very same system kicks in today when the boss shouts at you or the bus is caught in traffic when you are already late for an appointment. The hormones that prepare us to run away or fight are still released but neither situation requires a physical response. This leaves the body in an unbalanced, uncomfortable state. If the increased levels of adrenaline and other chemicals the body produces in response to a perceived threat are not used to fuel a physical reaction, the high levels of these hormones racing around the body can start to cause physical damage. Most people are aware that perpetually high levels of stress play a significant part in the development of heart disease. Scientists have now also found that high levels of cortisol, a key hormone released by the body during times of stress, can also affect the brain.

Post-traumatic stress disorder (PTSD) is a neuropsychiatric condition that affects people who have been through a very traumatic experience. They can be troubled by vivid flashbacks to the incident for many years afterwards. They also have elevated levels of cortisol in their blood, months and sometimes years after the event. It is as if the body has been unable to reset itself back to normal levels and it keeps the individual in a perpetual state of readiness to confront danger. MRI studies have shown that, over time, these high levels of cortisol begin to damage parts of the brain, particularly the hippocampi, brain structures that are critical in the formation of new memories.

Although chronic stress has a negative impact on memory function, acute stress appears to have the opposite effect. Numerous studies have shown that when people are under intense pressure they are actually better at learning new information and committing it to their long-term store, particularly if it has an emotional component. This is why people are often able to give detailed accounts of highly stressful events, for example if they witness an accident or are involved in a disaster. Many say it was as if the event occurred in slow motion, such was the vivid detail they could recall afterwards. This is sometimes called 'flashbulb memory' – as if the memory has been caught and captured on camera, such is its clarity.

Flashbulb memories: where were you then . . .?

Flashbulb memories are formed by a special biological memory mechanism, different from normal memory processes. The mechanism is only triggered by exceptional events. Immense surprise is also often a key characteristic. Personal flashbulb memories are usually centred on births, deaths and accidents. A number of events have been responsible for collective flashbulb memories, including the assassination of John F. Kennedy, the death of Diana, Princess of Wales, and the terrorist attacks of September 11, 2001, in the USA. Flashbulb memories are very robust and resistant to forgetting. The most enduring detail of a flashbulb memory is where you were when something happened. While the vividness and detail of flashbulb memories in people with Alzheimer's Disease does eventually fade, where they were when the flashbulb memory was formed is normally the last thing to go.

Unsurprisingly, there is a downside to the brain diverting all its available resources to consolidating new memories when you are under stress. The retrieval part of the memory system becomes far less efficient. It's much harder to recall something you already know when you are under pressure than when you are not. This will be familiar to anyone who has ever had a bad attack of 'exam nerves'.

Even if it were possible, it is undesirable to eliminate stress entirely from our lives. At the right level, stress hormones can make us feel excited, even exhilarated. This is why young children just can't seem to keep still when they are excited. Their bodies react physically to the increased energy released by the stress hormones. As adults we learn to suppress this natural physical response. Christmas, holidays and weddings are all associated with an increase in stress hormones, but we usually experience the changes within our bodies in response to these events as anticipatory excitement (for the most part at least – although it's easy to tip into feelings of rising panic, even on these happy occasions). The key to stress management is getting the balance just right.

Managing stress

There is much you can do to reduce the physical stress on your body. Maintaining a healthy lifestyle with a good balanced diet has become the modern-day mantra to help us avoid cancer and heart disease. The fact is, a fit, healthy body is an advantage for every human endeavour. Researchers in Sweden have recently found that people who are overweight in middle age increase their risk of developing Alzheimer's Disease by 70 per cent compared to those with a healthy Body Mass Index (BMI).

It is your reaction to a stressor that determines whether or not you become stressed by it. We are all very different in what we find stressful on a day-to-day basis. Some people seem to be able to shrug off minor arguments while others let the hurt fester for days. Some people daydream their way through a slow-moving queue while others become increasingly irate as every minute ticks by. Individual differences in the ways in which we respond to these potentially stressful situations are due to a unique mix of our genetic make-up, personality and things we have learnt along the way. Learning effective stress management will therefore be a very individual process. An appreciation that it is your reaction to an event that causes stress, *not* the event itself, that is intrinsically stressful is the first step along the way. Finding new ways to respond to events you naturally perceive as stressful can be difficult. Sometimes it involves undoing a lifetime of learning. There are many self-help books available on stress management and some are better than others. Meditation, relaxation techniques and learning to approach and think about situations in a different way can all be effective ways of managing stress. Finding an approach that you believe in, and feel comfortable with, will go a long way to reducing the stress in your life generally and will help to maximize the beneficial effects and minimize the detrimental effects that stress can have on memory function.

Anxiety and memory

Anxiety and stress are closely related. While stress comes from your reaction to something that makes you feel frustrated, anxiety is a feeling of unease and fear that occurs in the absence of an obvious, immediate trigger. A state of chronic anxiety often results from repeated exposure to multiple stressors. One simple rule of thumb for distinguishing between stress and anxiety is to look at the order of thoughts in relation to feelings. In anxiety, the unpleasant feelings often precede the thoughts that go with them. People with chronic anxiety often feel bad and then mentally search around for the thing that is making them feel anxious. Having found something to peg the feelings on, they can find it hard to feel better, as the feeling remains even when the apparent trigger issue has been resolved. Anxiety Disorder is a medical condition that occurs when anxiety levels become so elevated that they begin to interfere with people's lives. Memory problems are a diagnostic feature of the condition. Anxiety disorders can be treated with cognitive behavioural therapy (CBT) and sometimes medication is used to reset the brain chemistry.

Worry is a huge drain on the brain's resources, leaving little reserve for other functions. Raised levels of anxiety have a devastating effect on working memory, the system that temporarily holds several pieces of information in your mind and allows you to manipulate them to solve problems or make connections. A deficient working memory impacts almost every area of cognition. If you are unable to hold information and work with it at the same time, this will have a significant impact on your ability to take in and understand new information and plan and make decisions. As proficiency in these tasks decreases so anxiety increases even further as people begin to worry even more, and so a vicious cycle is created, with greater anxiety leading to even greater memory difficulties.

To reduce the impact of anxiety on memory function this vicious cycle must be broken. CBT is an effective method with proven results in this area. Your GP can refer you to your local Improving Access to Psychological Therapies (IAPT) service with therapists who are skilled in breaking these vicious cycles.

Mood and memory

Depression is the most prevalent mental health disorder in the UK. Almost 20 per cent of the population will experience a clinically significant episode of depression at some times in their lives. Rates of depression are currently so high that the World Health Organization (WHO) has ranked the condition as the single most burdensome disease in the world in middle-aged people, in terms of years of total disability. Depression is also highly recurrent; three out of four sufferers will experience more than one episode in their lifetime.

In addition to low mood, memory difficulties and problems concentrating are core diagnostic features of depression. They are part and parcel of the condition. Studies have shown that people with depression find it difficult to sustain sufficient attention to complete cognitive tasks. However, they find it much easier than healthy individuals to maintain their attention on negative thoughts about themselves. Researchers have shown that these negative thoughts hog the mental resources that depressed people need to function effectively. It is no surprise, therefore, that people with depression experience significant memory problems in everyday life.

Depression doesn't only reduce memory capacity: there is also evidence that the condition interferes with what people remember. People with depression appear to pay particular attention to negative information and are not able to properly process positive experiences. In laboratory tests where people are given lists of random words to memorize, depressed people tend to remember 10 per cent more negative words than positive ones. In real life, they tend to remember events that are congruent with their mood. This bias doesn't just apply to new memories; when they are asked to remember events from the past, people who are depressed are able to recall negative information and events from their long-term memory store with ease, but have difficulties recalling more positive memories.

These changes in memory function are accompanied by changes in the brain. The hippocampi are particularly vulnerable to the neurotoxic effects of depression. The altered neurochemisty damages hippocampal neurons and causes the structures to shrink. The extent of the shrinkage is associated with the length of depression and the number of distinct episodes of depression experienced across a lifetime. The extent of the shrinkage is also correlated with the magnitude of associated memory problems. The smaller the hippocampi, the greater the memory problems, particularly in the learning of new information. Although some of the changes that cause the volume loss in the hippocampi are reversible, some studies have shown that the hippocampi of people who have only ever experienced one episode of depression remain smaller than those in people of a similar age who have never experienced the condition.

As with anxiety, memory problems are an integral part of having depression. They are not a side effect or a separate entity. Effective treatments in the form of psychological therapies and medications for clinical depression are available. Generally, as an individual's mood begins to lift after treatment so his or her memory problems subside, although some residual difficulties may always remain, particularly when it comes to taking in new information. Accepting that this is part of the condition is the first step to coping. Utilizing the strategies outlined in the earlier chapters of this book will help to reduce the nuisance of these difficulties.

8

Physical health and illness

Introduction

It is beyond the scope of this chapter to cover all of the effects that physical health can have on memory function. Some illnesses and their treatments can have a direct impact on brain function and memory difficulties may be a key diagnostic feature or a well-known side effect of the treatment. In other conditions, memory problems may arise indirectly from the effects of pain, fever, fatigue and other general symptoms of just feeling unwell, particularly in chronic conditions. The purpose of this chapter is to highlight some of the most common physical conditions and medical treatments that can interfere with memory function. The list is by no means exhaustive, and if your condition isn't covered it doesn't mean that memory isn't affected. If you are worried about memory problems it's always helpful to start with a review of your physical health and any medications you may be taking.

The brain is the most complex and costly organ in the human body in terms of its energy demands. In newborn babies, the brain takes up nearly 90 per cent of the baby's energy. This decreases with age, but even in adults the brain uses 20 per cent of the body's energy. If the body is busy fighting off illness it can have a significant impact on the amount of energy available for the brain. In some infections, particularly those involving bacteria or parasites, body tissues are damaged and must be replaced, and this is a costly process in terms of the energy it requires. Many illnesses cause diarrhoea, which can severely limit the body's intake of nutrients, our source of energy. Some viruses use our cells to reproduce themselves at our expense, so energy is diverted to sustain them instead of us. Whenever you are ill, your body activates your immune system to fight off the illness. Again, this takes a lot of energy. It follows, then, that whenever you are under the weather, less energy may be available for your brain to function at its best. This has been demonstrated even in the common cold.

Memory and the common cold

In 2012 researchers from Cardiff University studied the effects of the common cold on the memory functions of 200 otherwise healthy young people aged between 18 and 30 years. All the volunteers were well at the beginning of the study when they completed the first set of memory tests. They returned to see the researchers when they next contracted a cold, and completed the tests again. The researchers made sure that the volunteers had a cold rather than flu or something more serious. They found that when the students had a cold they processed information far more slowly than when they were well. They were also slower at taking in new information.

While any kind of illness may have a temporarily dampening effect on optimal brain function, some conditions have a specific impact on memory function. Some of the most common are discussed below.

Diabetes

Diabetes and memory loss are closely linked. Memory function can be acutely affected in a hypoglycaemic attack (a hypo) when blood sugar levels drop too low and the brain does not get enough glucose to function effectively. There is not enough fuel to enable the brain cells (neurons) to effectively communicate with other and so, one by one, the cognitive systems start to shut down. If blood sugars are not normalized, the person may eventually slip into a coma. Poorly controlled diabetes with perpetually high levels of blood sugar (hyperglycaemia) can also cause brain damage over time, which can lead to permanent difficulties in memory function. The hippocampi seem to be particularly vulnerable to damage in diabetes. Hippocampal shrinkage has been recorded in both elderly and young populations with type II diabetes.

People with diabetes are also at increased risk for both Alzheimer's Disease and vascular dementia. Amylin is a hormone expressed and secreted with insulin. It influences blood sugar levels, and when too much is secreted amylin deposits can build up and form plaques in the brain, similar to the amyloid plaques found in Alzheimer's Disease. When amylin is over-produced and is not cleared normally from the system in someone with diabetes, the build-up can lead to the loss of brain cells and a progressive deterioration in cognitive function.

Vitamin B12 deficiency

Humans rely on Vitamin B12 to function properly. When levels within the body are only slightly lower than they should be, people can begin to experience exhaustion, depression and memory problems. If it is untreated, chronic Vitamin B12 deficiency can cause severe and irreversible damage to the brain and nervous system and the associated memory problems can resemble a dementia, as they become increasingly severe. The longer someone has the deficiency, the more likely it is that permanent damage will occur. It's not difficult to include sources of Vitamin B12 in a normal carnivorous diet, as it is found in many animal products, including meat, poultry, fish, seafood, eggs and dairy products. It is also usually added to fortified breakfast cereals. Most people with a Vitamin B12 deficiency cannot absorb the vitamin from their diet for some reason, rather than because they are not eating enough of the correct foods. There are many medical reasons for mal-absorption, including pernicious anaemia, surgical resection of part of the gut, infestation by parasites and rare hereditary conditions. Mal-absorption can also occur in chronic alcoholism. Fortunately Vitamin B12 deficiency can be treated and memory problems can often be reversed following treatment if no permanent brain damage has occurred. Even if neuronal damage has occurred, treatment in the form of injections, sprays, patches or pills normally stops the progression of memory decline.

Thyroid disorders

Thyroid disorders are relatively common in the general population with some studies suggesting that about 8 per cent of the population over the age of 50 may have an under-active thyroid (hypothyroidism). Symptoms of hypothyroidism can include fatigue, weight gain, poor concentration and memory problems. These problems can come on very gradually and people may live with them for many years before the problem is diagnosed. Fortunately hypothyroidism can be easily diagnosed with a simple blood test and the treatment involves taking a simple supplement to ensure the body has enough thyroxin to function properly, with no side effects at the correct dose. Generally the memory problems associated with hypothyroidism fully resolve following appropriate treatment.

Post-operative cognitive dysfunction

'Post-operative cognitive dysfunction' (POCD) is the term used to describe changes in memory function that can occur after an anaesthetic. It is common to experience mild memory difficulties in the immediate post-operative period as the anaesthetic wears off and strong painkillers are administered, both of which have a powerful influence on brain function. However, some people experience more long-term problems with memory function after surgery, problems that persist after the operation. POCD was originally identified in patients who had undergone lengthy cardiac surgery, but more recently doctors have recognized that it can happen after other types of surgery too. The risk of developing long-term memory problems following an anaesthetic increases with age and the length and number of surgical procedures. It is also more common in patients who develop post-operative infections. Some studies have suggested that people who develop POCD are at increased risk of developing dementia later on.

One study found that approximately half of all people over the age of 65 who underwent general anaesthesia had memory problems for at least 24 hours after surgery. One third of the patients still had some memory problems when they were discharged from hospital. The causes of this memory loss are not clear and there are no proven treatments or prevention strategies, but scientists are working on modified anaesthetics that block some of the neuro-receptors in the brain that are thought to contribute to memory deficits. POCD is rare after minor procedures that are conducted under light sedation and it is unusual for memory problems to persist in younger people.

Chemotherapy

'Chemo fog' or 'chemo brain' refers to the mental fog that many people experience during and after they have undergone chemotherapy for cancer. Common difficulties include an inability to sustain concentration, word-finding difficulties, slowed-up thinking and trouble multitasking. These symptoms can be extremely distressing and hard to cope with, particularly as they tend to come hard on the heels of all the other difficulties a diagnosis of cancer brings. Estimates of the percentage of people who suffer 'chemo brain' vary widely and range from 15 to 70 per cent in medical studies. This percentage depends largely on how 'chemo brain' is defined and how the cognitive problems are measured. 'Chemo brain' appears to be more common after some types of treatments than others. Many people may feel 'foggy' immediately after a chemotherapy treatment, but fewer report problems that persist after the treatment has finished.

Brain-imaging studies have shown that some of the parts of the brain that are involved with memory appear to shrink slightly following some kinds of chemotherapy. The volume loss also appears to be more common in people who undergo high doses of chemotherapy. Some forms of chemotherapy are known to cause nerve damage. These drugs are evolving all the time and current research is focused on ensuring maximum benefit while protecting brain function and minimizing cognitive side effects.

It is not only the type and dose of chemotherapy that determines whether it will be associated with cognitive problems. Genetic differences may make some people more susceptible than others. The APOE gene is linked to Alzheimer's Disease. If someone has the E4 version of this gene, that person may also have a higher risk of developing long-term memory problems following chemotherapy.

It is important to remember that not all memory problems in those with cancer are caused by chemotherapy. One study found a similar level of memory problems in a group of people with cancer who didn't undergo chemotherapy. Memory problems can be caused or exacerbated by many features of having cancer, including the cancer itself, exhaustion, sleep problems, depression, stress and anxiety. Other drugs used as part of treatment, such as steroids, anti-nausea medications, drugs used for surgery or pain medicines, may also be responsible for memory problems in these groups.

Psychiatric conditions

There is an increasing overlap in our understanding of psychiatric and neurological conditions. Sophisticated scans have revealed structural and chemical abnormalities in the brains of people who suffer psychiatric illness, and the lines of distinction between the two medical specialties have become increasingly blurred as a result. It follows then that the disturbances in thought and behaviour that accompany psychiatric illness often have a significant impact on memory function. It is also the case that external strategies tend to work better than internal ones in this group. However, when behaviour and thoughts are very disturbed, for example in acute psychiatric conditions, it is often difficult to implement methodical routines and, as with neurological conditions, an acceptance of memory problems as part of the condition is necessary.

Coping with memory problems in these contexts

You probably already track the primary symptoms of your condition for your doctor; it will also help if you track your memory problems. Keep a diary of when you notice problems. You may notice a pattern emerging if you note down what was happening when the memory problems occurred. This includes details about when the information should have been processed *and* when you were trying to recall it or realized that you had forgotten something. It may be that memory lapses are more common at certain times of the day or just after you have taken your medicine. Forewarned is forearmed; if a pattern does emerge you can start to plan. You may be able to avoid putting yourself in situations where you will be expected to take in a lot of information at vulnerable times or, if you can't avoid them, you can make contingency plans (take someone else with you or make extra-careful notes). It's good practice to make a list of all the questions you may have or points that you want to get across before a meeting or appointment, and perfectly OK to take the list along with you.

Summary

Physical health affects brain function. Many common chronic conditions have a direct impact on memory function. Many medical treatments can also have an adverse effect on brain function. Sometimes the effect is temporary, while in other conditions the impact can be permanent and or progressive. Accepting the fact that memory problems are part of a diagnosis and/or treatment is the first step to reducing the nuisance of memory difficulties. In the majority of cases the most effective strategies involve the outsourcing of memory functions to external agencies rather than attempts to boost brain power with mnemonic tricks. The external agencies can be physical (diaries, calendars, notes), digital (phone apps, alarms, etc.), environmental (the development of set routines) and social (the help of friends and family). Although these strategies are all designed to reduce the nuisance rather than restore function, it is also possible to maximize the underlying brain function with the appropriate diet and exercise. These mechanisms are discussed in Chapter 10.

9

Neurological conditions

Every neurological condition has the potential to affect memory function since, by definition, every neurological condition is the result of brain dysfunction at some level or other. Sometimes this dysfunction may fluctuate and be temporary, for example in certain types of Multiple Sclerosis (MS) and epilepsy. In other conditions the underlying damage or dysfunction may be stable but permanent, such as a traumatic brain injury or a stroke. In progressive conditions, memory problems increase over time as the disease runs its course. Although neurologists have many drugs at their disposal to treat neurological conditions, any drug that acts on the brain also has the potential to further disrupt memory function.

There are three groups of factors that influence memory function in neurological disorders. The first group includes factors that are fixed and can't be changed. This includes the nature of the underlying brain pathology and where it is in the brain. Your age at the onset of symptoms can also have an impact on the extent of associated memory difficulties. As a rule, younger brains tend to adapt better to damage and trauma than older ones. The course of the disease will also have an impact on memory function over time. This is the second factor that will influence memory function. In epilepsy, an episode of status epilepticus (a very prolonged seizure that will not stop), repeated generalized seizures or multiple head injuries can lead to stepwise increases in memory difficulties. Neurosurgical interventions in other conditions can also have an irreversible impact on memory function.

The third group of factors that influence memory function in neurological conditions includes remediable factors. These are factors that you may be able to modify to reduce the impact they have. They include medications, mood and lifestyle factors ranging from diet to quality of sleep. With medications it is often a question of finding the right balance between efficacy (effectiveness) and side effects when it comes to managing any exacerbation of memory difficulties associated with the drugs. This is particularly the case with antiepileptic drugs. If you suspect that your medications are exacerbating your memory problems, talk to your neurologist, who may be able to adjust the dose or try a different combination to minimize these effects.

Other neurological conditions

If you have been diagnosed with a neurological condition it is likely that your memory will be affected. It would be possible to write separate books on the specific cognitive problems commonly seen in each and every different neurological condition. Much useful information and advice can be found on the websites of the charities and organizations that deal with each separate condition. Different conditions are associated with different patterns of memory problems. Some conditions affect new learning, while others may make it difficult to recall events from the past. If you have been diagnosed with a neurological illness, talk to your neurologist about the typical pattern of memory difficulties associated with your condition. Specialist neuropsychological assessments can be used to find out exactly where the normal memory procedures are breaking down in each individual. Neuropsychologists use these patterns to devise packages of tailored strategies to help. However, there are no magic answers to a poor memory caused by brain damage or disease.

Acceptance of the memory problems as part and parcel of the condition is a key part of any rehabilitation (see page 65). The most effective strategies to lessen the nuisance of a poor memory in people with a neurological condition are primarily based on the outsourcing of tasks that would normally be done by the brain to physical media (such as notes, calendars, diaries, mobile phone apps and alarms). The use of the internal strategies that strengthen memory processes are generally less effective in people who have an underlying structural reason for their memory problems than in the general population.

Coping with memory problems in these contexts

When memory problems are due to a neurological or psychiatric condition, acceptance is a key part of coping. Many people can accept the physical limitations their condition may impose, but struggle to accept that memory difficulties are also an integral part of the disorder. The struggle for psychological control over these problems may be futile and even counterproductive if the memory-processing parts of the brain have been irrevocably damaged by disease or trauma. However, once you have accepted that you have memory problems there are a number of things you can do that can dramatically reduce the nuisance they cause in everyday life. The first is to tell other people about the situation. These can include friends, family and your doctor. Sometimes just telling someone what you are going through can relieve the burden and provide reassurance that you are not going mad.

More importantly, you may be able to enlist people's help. You may not have difficulties asking for help with mobility, or for someone to read letters for you if your vision is poor, but you may feel uncomfortable asking for help when it comes to memory. It is OK to ask friends and family for help in this area too. They may be able to help with daily tasks to cut down on distractions and allow you to save mental energy and focus on just one thing, or they may be able to accompany you to an important appointment, where two heads will be better than one in taking in new information.

It may not just be a question of telling people about your memory problems: it can be a two-way conversation. Sometimes it's helpful to ask family members whether they have noticed any changes in your memory. You may be reassured that your problems are not as bad as you think, or they may have noticed some things you haven't and could have some helpful suggestions. For instance, your children may have noticed that when you are rushed you have more trouble finding things or don't take in information properly (they may even be exploiting this!). You can address this by budgeting extra time for tasks and asking people to drop you an email or leave a note or text reminder if they have asked you to do something when you are in the middle of doing something else and are not in a position to create a memory jog yourself.

Having told people about your problems and enlisted their help where possible, the final piece of outsourcing involves the development of routines. This may involve some reorganization in your life, and again your friends and family can help. Choose a specific place for things you frequently lose and practise putting them there each time you come in. Set up and follow set routines for the regular tasks you complete to try to ensure that you can focus on one thing at a time.

While memory problems associated with neurological disorders are generally intractable and you will need to rely on external aids to reduce the nuisance, following the advice on diet and exercise in the next chapter will ensure that you maximize the physical potential of your brain. It is also the case that elevated levels of anxiety and depression are very common in people with neurological and other psychiatric conditions, and reducing these levels may well have a beneficial effect on memory function.

10

Diet and exercise

It is well established that people who exercise regularly live longer, are less likely to develop heart disease and cancer and are less depressed than people who live sedentary lifestyles. Exercise is good for us. Aerobic exercise is particularly good for us. Any physical activity that gets our heart beating faster makes us fitter. The more often this activity is repeated, the fitter we get, and the fitter our bodies are, the better equipped they are to fight almost every disease or ailment we will ever encounter. This is not to say fit people don't get ill – they do – but they are less likely to develop serious health problems, and even when they do develop them they tend to survive for longer. This makes sense. Our bodies and brains work best when the amount of fat we have is in the correct proportion to our lean tissue (muscle tissue without fat) and our heart and lungs are strong and able to supply and deliver the oxygen we need throughout our body. Although your brain is only about 2 per cent of your body mass, it uses up approximately 20 per cent of your oxygen consumption every day. It needs the right fuel to function effectively. This is influenced to some extent by diet, but the delivery system also has to be effective. To view brain function as separate from other vital organs when it comes to fitness is a mistake. Your brain health and function is closely linked to your physical condition. It follows that exercise and physical fitness have a significant effect on memory function.

As explained in Chapter 1, the hippocampi are two seahorse-shaped structures in the brain that play a crucial role in laying down new memories. Unfortunately they shrink as we get older and, as they do so, memory problems increase. It's possible to measure the size of the hippocampi using sophisticated MRI scans. Scientists have found that these structures are larger in adults who are physically fit.

71

Walk yourself to a bigger brain

A group of researchers from the USA wanted to find out whether it was possible for unfit people to increase the size of their hippocampi by doing exercise. They scanned 120 older adults, aged between 60 and 70, and measured their hippocampi. Half of the subjects were then enrolled on an exercise programme. They began by walking for five minutes a day and then gradually increased the time over a period of four weeks until they were walking for 40 minutes, three days a week. The other half of the group exercised for a similar length of time in stretching and toning classes. One year later the researchers measured the size of the hippocampi in the two groups again. The people who had completed the exercise training had increased their hippocampal volumes by 2 per cent, effectively reversing age-related volume loss by one to two years. These volume increases were also accompanied by improvements on memory tests. The researchers concluded that taking up exercise in older age had a significant impact on both brain structure and memory function.

It's never too early to benefit from exercise from a memory perspective. Exercise in mid-life is also associated with a decreased risk of developing dementia in older age. Some studies have estimated that the risks are reduced by up to one third. Walking just one mile a day (perhaps to the local shops and back) can make all the difference.

Obesity

The rise in obesity in the UK over the past 20 years has been phenomenal. Obesity has now reached epidemic proportions, with 60 per cent of the UK adult population classified as overweight. One in four adults is obese (i.e. has a BMI of over 30). Over 30,000 people die in the UK every year from causes that are directly attributable to obesity. This means that obesity-related deaths account for 6 per cent of all recorded deaths every year. Sadly, one third of these people die before the age of 65. Obesity in middle age is not only associated with an increased risk of developing dementia in old

age; middle-aged people who are obese have more memory problems than those of a similar age and background who are a healthy
weight. They also have smaller hippocampi. Where you carry your
excess weight also has a significant influence on hippocampal
health. One study found that central obesity (classic 'apple' shapes
who carry their weight around their middles) is particularly damaging for the hippocampi. Studies have shown that the larger
your waist to hip ratio is, the smaller your hippocampi tend to be.
Apple-shaped individuals are at increased risk of developing cancer,
cardiovascular disease and memory problems. Unfortunately we
can't choose where we store excess weight, but if you are apple-
shaped and tend to gain weight around your middle, conserving
your hippocampal health is yet another reason to keep your weight
under control.

Obesity is also associated with a much faster age-related decline
in memory efficiency. In 2012, doctors reported the results of a
study that had tracked a series of over 6,000 people across a ten-year
period. The study recruits were given three memory and cognitive
tests over the course of the decade. The decline in performance
on the tests was 22 per cent faster in the people who were obese
compared to those with a normal healthy weight.

The good news is that these memory problems reduce (along
with BMI) when people follow a diet that results in successful
weight loss. Scientists in Sweden tested a group of 20 overweight
women on memory tests before assigning them to two different
kinds of diet. One was the 'caveman diet', a diet based upon foods
that our early ancestors would have eaten: nuts and seeds and no
processed foods. The second group followed a standard, low-fat,
balanced diet. Both groups lost weight and both performed much
better on the memory tests after six months of successful dieting.
Sophisticated MRI scans also demonstrated positive changes in the
blood flow in the brains of the women while they were completing
the memory tests. The message from the exercise and obesity
studies seems to be clear. Weight loss (however it is achieved) and
increased fitness levels have physical effects on the brain that actually improve memory function, even in old age.

Diet

As evidenced above, any diet that results in weight loss in the overweight has a good chance of improving memory function, but do the foods we eat actually have a direct impact on brain function? There has been a lot of marketing of 'superfoods' in recent years with some remarkable claims made for some. Blueberries in particular have been linked to an incredible range of health benefits. While much of what is touted on the internet is hype, with a very thin or non-existent evidence base, there may be something behind the claims that blueberries forestall or even reverse age-related deteriorations in brain cells, as well as the problems in memory function these cause. Blueberries exert their beneficial effects in two ways. They appear to lower inflammation and alter the signalling involved in neuronal communication. These benefits are not just limited to blueberries. Flavonoids (or bioflavonoids) – from the Latin word *flavus*, meaning yellow – are a class of plant compound. They are present in a number of colourful foods. A number of studies have suggested that diets that incorporate flavonoid-rich foods, such as blueberries, green tea, cocoa and ginkgo biloba, can lead to reversals of age-related deficits on tests of spatial memory and learning. Much of this evidence come from animal studies, where scientists have timed how long it has taken rats fed with blueberries and other flavonoids to learn a maze, compared with rats on a normal rat diet.

Can two cups of cocoa a day keep memory problems at bay?

In August 2013 a small-scale study, primarily reporting a way of measuring blood flow to the brain, hit the international headlines. The *Daily Mail* went with 'Drinking hot chocolate could prevent Alzheimers' while the *Sun* ran with '2 cups of hot chocolate a night could fight dementia'. As is often the way with these things, the actual conclusions from the study were more complicated than the news reporting suggested, and the study wasn't actually even about dementia. The researchers had set out to see whether cocoa with a high flavonoid content was more effective than cocoa with a low flavonoid content in improving blood flow to the brain in people who had high blood pressure and/or diabetes. They didn't find any differences between the two types of cocoa, but they did find that in the people who started out with particularly poor blood flows, blood flow was increased and cognitive performance was improved after they had been drinking cocoa twice a day for a month. There was no difference for people who had normal blood flow to begin with. The message seems to be that cocoa might help to improve processing speed if blood flow to the brain is compromised by vascular disease or diabetes.

There has yet to be a definitive study in people proving the beneficial effects of flavonoids, but this is currently a very active area of research: the evidence to date is promising and suggests that it may be an avenue worth pursuing. In the meantime, the only harm associated with eating blueberries on a regular basis is likely to be to your wallet, so it may be worth a try. The same can be said for cocoa, but be careful that the extra calories associated with the milk and sugar don't lead you to pile on the pounds or this will soon outweigh any potential benefits.

While the brain-boosting power of some foods remains an intriguing possibility, it is clear that some diets are associated with accelerated damage to brain cells, in particular the brain cells in the hippocampi – the brain structures that are critical for forming new memories. A high intake of saturated fats and simple carbohydrates is not only linked with the development of obesity and an increased risk of Alzheimer's Disease, but is also correlated with biological changes in the hippocampus well before the development of Alzheimer's Disease. Some scientists have even argued that the hippocampal dysfunction caused by this kind of diet interferes with our ability to stop ourselves from responding to environmental cues associated with food, ultimately making us eat more than we need when food is plentiful, and so a vicious cycle is created. The more saturated fat and sugar we eat, the more likely we are to lose touch with feelings of hunger and satiety. We then begin to eat in response to external cues, primarily the availability of food and the amount on our plates.

It is beyond the scope of this book to discuss the general health benefits of a balanced diet. Much advice about healthy eating and recommended guidelines for sugar and fat is available on the UK NHS website (see 'Useful addresses and resources' at the back of this book for further information). Many people are already aware of what constitutes a healthy diet – it's sticking to it that is the problem. This is partly due to the long-term nature of dietary changes required for success and the lack of immediate results. However, when it comes to memory function, many people do report a 'clearing' of their minds within just a few days of a low-fat, low-carbohydrate regime. As with the blueberries, you have nothing to lose (except weight) and everything to gain with this approach.

Summary

Physical exercise and a healthy diet maximize physical health. They also optimize brain function. Exercise can actually increase the size of the hippocampi and reverse age-related decline. On the other hand, a diet high in saturated fat and sugar contributes to hippocampal dysfunction and significantly increases the risk of Alzheimer's Disease in later life. If you are serious about maximizing your memory function, getting your physical health right is just as important as all the memory strategies in this book. Although it's a lifelong commitment, the cognitive benefits of making changes in these areas of your life can sometimes be felt within a few days.

11

Hormonal changes

The correct balance of oestrogen, progesterone, testosterone and thyroid hormones is as essential for maintaining cognitive functions as food-based nutrients are for keeping the body working properly. The concentrations of these hormones are often higher in the brain than they are in the bloodstream. Some brain cells actually produce their own supply. It follows, then, that hormone imbalances can have a dramatic effect on brain function. There are a number of stages in a woman's life where hormone levels are in flux, all of which can be associated with memory loss and poor concentration. This chapter examines the role that hormones can play in memory difficulties during the menstrual cycle, during pregnancy and childbirth, and during and after the menopause.

Memory and the menstrual cycle

Many women experience regular changes in mood at certain times in their menstrual cycle. There is a large amount of evidence that suggests that memory functions also fluctuate across the menstrual cycle. Women tend to perform better on tests of verbal fluency and on tasks that require fine motor skill in the mid-phase of their cycle, while they perform better on tests of spatial ability during the menstrual phase. These fluctuations in cognitive performance are correlated with the fluctuating levels of estradiol (an important ovarian sex hormone) throughout the menstrual cycle. Levels of estradiol are correlated positively with scores on tests of verbal fluency and negatively with scores on tests of spatial ability. Although these patterns are evident in group studies, there is considerable individual variation in the extent to which people notice these fluctuations in their everyday life. Just as some people experience large mood swings prior to the onset of a period while others rarely notice any changes, so the influence of normal hormonal fluctuations on memory function can vary. Some people seem to be more susceptible than others. Keeping a diary of memory lapses may help you to identify any cyclical aspects to memory problems that you may be experiencing. If a cyclical pattern does emerge, you may be able to arrange important work–life commitments to avoid the times when you may be more likely to struggle.

Pregnancy and childbirth

Memory changes associated with pregnancy and childbirth have received a lot of attention in recent years. Many studies have found that pregnant women and new mothers perform more poorly on memory tests than women of a similar age who are not pregnant or who have not given birth. Some have argued that these memory problems are simply due to the stress and sleep deprivation associated with pregnancy and looking after a new baby. The physical stress of pregnancy on the body is huge. Remember the studies of the effect of the common cold on memory function in Chapter 8? If the metabolic cost of fighting off a simple cold causes a reduction in memory proficiency, it is no surprise that growing a new human being takes a huge toll.

However, there is also an increasing body of evidence that suggests that the dramatic hormonal changes that occur in pregnancy and childbirth also have a direct impact on brain function, particularly memory abilities. Again, some women seem more susceptible to these changes than others. For most women, memory problems that come on during the final trimester of pregnancy tend to resolve over the first year of their child's life. However, there is some evidence to suggest that these problems may persist longer in women who undergo a very traumatic birth, where levels of the stress hormone cortisol are raised for a prolonged period, possibly causing some damage to hippocampal cells.

Memory problems following childbirth are difficult to cope with. There is so much new information to take in and new mothers are often in a perpetual state of exhaustion and anxiety. Accepting that these problems are common and finding support from other new mothers can be helpful. As with other forms of memory difficulty, setting up clear routines, accepting all the help you can get and not expecting too much of yourself, particularly in the early days, will also ease the burden on your memory until things normalize again.

Menopause and post-menopause

The menopause signals the end of menstruation. In the UK the average age for the menopause is 52. A menopause that occurs before the age of 45 is classified as premature. As the oestrogen levels decrease, menstrual periods become less frequent and many women experience a variety of physical symptoms including hot flushes (sometimes called 'personal summers' or 'tropical moments'), night sweats, insomnia (sometimes exacerbated by vivid nightmares), itchy skin and mood swings. Women often notice an increase in memory problems during the menopause.

Jean's story
I hit 50 and thought I was going mad. Suddenly it felt as if my brain was stuffed with cotton wool. I would try to read the newspaper and ended up just staring at a page and realizing five minutes later that nothing was going in. I would go into a room and have no idea what I went in for. I'd start a conversation and then completely forget what I was about to say. My children joked about me having dementia and I would go along with the joke, but inside I was really scared. Although there is no family history I'd convinced myself that I had Alzheimer's Disease.

The risks and benefits of hormone replacement therapy

Studies have shown that hormone replacement therapy (HRT) can have a beneficial effect on memory function in some women, but the timing is critical. If HRT is initiated seamlessly with the onset of a natural menopause, and it is taken for two to three years, it is associated with a decreased risk of memory problems in later life. Some studies suggest that these protective effects can last up to 10–15 years after the HRT has been stopped. However, when HRT is started in older women who have already been through the menopause it seems to be associated with a higher risk of dementia. There appears to be a 'healthy cell bias' in the action of oestrogen on the brain. When healthy neurons are exposed to oestrogen it has a beneficial effect on their survival, but it seems to exacerbate the demise of already compromised neurons.

The surgical removal of the uterus and ovaries is often performed in premenopausal women for the treatment of benign gynaecological disorders. This effectively deprives them of several years of oestrogen exposure. Studies comparing women who received HRT immediately after these procedures with women who didn't found that the HRT appears to protect memory skills. Long-term studies have found that women who undergo this kind of surgery but who then take HRT until the age of 50 (the approximate time of the natural menopause) had no increased risk of cognitive impairment or dementia and their memory skills were comparable to women who had undergone a natural menopause at 50.

Summary

Hormones have a direct impact on cognitive function. The natural fluctuations associated with the menstrual cycle influence memory function. Memory can also be significantly affected during pregnancy, following childbirth and during the menopause. Knowing that this is common can help people cope. People who take HRT at the time of the menopause tend to have fewer memory problems than those who don't, but there is a lot of individual variation in the response to both the menopause and HRT. Some people sail through, some really suffer.

The evidence seems to indicate that if HRT is started at the onset of the menopause and is then taken for a few years, it may provide some protection against the development of significant memory problems in later life. In people who undergo an early menopause, taking HRT until a natural menopause would have occurred also appears to provide some protection of memory abilities. However, there are no benefits to taking HRT in later life and some studies have indicated that taking HRT over the age of 65, or starting it well after the menopause has ended, can be harmful. The decision to take HRT should be discussed carefully with your doctor as the risks and benefits extend well beyond the cognitive sphere.

12

Normal age-related cognitive decline

Introduction

Although we legally classify anyone over the age of 18 as an adult, the human brain doesn't fully mature until the mid-twenties. The frontal lobes (the regions of the brain behind your forehead) are the last parts to mature. The frontal lobes are responsible for most of the characteristics that make us an adult, including the ability to plan and sequence actions, weigh up evidence and make decisions, and anticipate both the immediate and the wider consequences of our actions. The frontal lobes also play an important role in helping us to infer the mental state of other people and reflect upon, and develop insight into, our own behaviour. The reason children and teenagers are so bad at these things is because their frontal lobes haven't matured yet. This fact has even been used as a defence against murder charges levelled at young people in the USA.

The case of Christopher Simmons

Christopher Simmons was a 17-year-old schoolboy when he was charged with the murder of Shirley Crook, a 46-year-old housewife from Missouri, in 1993. Mrs Crook died as the result of a shockingly brutal and callous attack. When he was arrested, Simmons quickly confessed to the murder. The court was presented with clear evidence of premeditation and heard from witnesses who said he had bragged about the crime afterwards. The jury found him guilty and recommended the death sentence, partly because of the senseless violence of the attack. Simmons appealed and the case went to the Supreme Court, where evidence was heard from neuroscientists who argued that, at 17, Simmons' brain had not sufficiently matured to make him fully culpable for the crime. Although there was clear evidence of premeditation, Simmons was not deemed to be wholly able to appreciate the full consequences of his actions. His sentence was commuted to a life term. As a result of this case, the Supreme Court of the United States determined that it was unconstitutional to impose capital punishment for crimes committed while under the age of 18. The decision overturned statutes in 25 American states that had previously set the penalty at a younger age.

Although brain maturation takes over two decades, some functions have already started to deteriorate by the time we reach 30. Age-related decline in cognitive function tends to follow a set pattern, with some abilities preserved and others going downhill at various gradients over the course of our lives. These changes are thought to have some evolutionary advantages, with wisdom and knowledge superseding physical prowess as we get older.

Psychologists divide cognitive functions into different domains. There are four main abilities that comprise intellectual function – the way in which we understand and interact with the world.

Verbal comprehension

Verbal comprehension is a measure of how well you can understand and use language. This can include the extent of your vocabulary and also how well you understand and can express abstract concepts. Verbal comprehension also includes general knowledge about the world. As a rule, these abilities continue to develop throughout life, even into the seventh decade. Even in very old age (over the age of 80) these abilities are generally preserved and are not subject to marked age-related declines in healthy individuals. Traditionally these abilities are classed as wisdom, hence the idea that they are greater in the old than the young.

Perceptual reasoning

Perceptual reasoning is the ability to spot visual patterns and make sense of three-dimensional relationships. Reading a map upside down or being able to complete a Rubik's Cube requires good perceptual reasoning skills. If you have well-developed perceptual reasoning skills you will be able to look at an IKEA self-assembly instruction sheet and immediately see in your mind's eye how the pieces fit together. Although people with good verbal comprehension skills also tend to be good at these tasks, the two things don't always go together. Sometimes people can be brilliant in one area and hopeless in another. Genes probably play a large role in determining your individual strengths and weaknesses across the cognitive domains. Unlike verbal dexterity, perceptual reasoning appears to peak early in life and proficiency remains relatively stable from the age of 16 to the mid-thirties. However, these abilities then begin a steady decline over the following decades into old age, with the steepest decline between the mid-forties to the mid-sixties.

When examining the effects of ageing on cognitive functions it is important to take into account your proficiency in your earlier life. If map reading has never been your forte, it's not surprising if you struggle to collapse or put up your new grandchild's super-slick, space-saving buggy when you first encounter it in your fifties.

Working memory

Working memory is the ability to hold a piece of information in your head and manipulate it at the same time. Mental arithmetic relies on working memory; you need to keep the figures in your head and manipulate them at the same time for success. We use working memory all the time to plan and make decisions, particularly when working on the logistics of any given situation. Working memory underpins many everyday tasks. Studies have shown that working memory skills are developed by the age of 18 and remain stable until the mid-fifties. They then begin to gradually deteriorate. Difficulties sustaining concentration and new difficulties in 'losing the thread' often begin to emerge in the mid-fifties. These difficulties are usually due to normal age-related declines in working memory.

Processing speed

Of the four principal intellectual domains, processing speed is the function that shows the most dramatic decline with age. Processing speed refers to the speed with which we can take in and react to information from the outside world. Studies of reaction time have shown that there is little change until around the age of 50 on simple tasks that just require someone to press a button as fast as possible in response to a given signal. However, when the task is made more complicated and an element of decision-making introduced (e.g. 'Hit the right-hand button when you see a blue circle on the screen'), slowed processing speeds become apparent as early as the late twenties. By the mid-fifties this slowing begins to manifest itself in everyday life. In busy environments, where there is a lot to take in, people may need information to be repeated, or they may miss key pieces of information if it is presented too quickly and they are still processing things that have been said earlier. In busy office environments and in meetings where the conversation is fast flowing and lots of ideas are being bounced around, slowed processing speed can be responsible for people missing key decisions and conversations. Finding ways to slow the rate of information is the most effective way of dealing with this normal age-related decline. This may include introducing a clear structure to office meetings and ensuring that they are chaired competently, and recapping after every topic has been discussed before moving on to the next one. These strategies work well if they are in your control. However, for most of us they are not.

If there is little you can do to slow the external flow of information, your next best bet is to outsource the recording of information as a back-up for your memory which will allow you to digest the details at your leisure. Dictaphones, Livescribe pens and effective note-taking may be the answer to reducing the embarrassment and nuisance slowed processing can cause in professional situations (see 'Useful addresses and resources' on page 117). In social situations this is usually less of an issue if you socialize with people of a similar age, as the conversation naturally adjusts to the common speed. However, it is beneficial to be aware of the gradual, natural decline in processing speed when talking to people older than yourself, even those without any obvious cognitive impairments, and to adjust the flow of information accordingly, providing additional back-ups in the form of repetition or written confirmations when appropriate.

Memory skills

It is also the case that memory skills naturally deteriorate with age. This deterioration affects both the learning of new material and, to a lesser extent, the recall of well-learnt information. Memory function declines gradually from middle age to the mid-sixties. However, after the age of 70, this decline accelerates even in otherwise healthy individuals. In the same way that our skin ages as we get older, these changes simply reflect the natural ageing process of the brain. As with all other aspects of ageing, there are significant individual differences in the rate and extent of decline. These will be dictated by your genes, your environment and your physical health (see Chapters 10 and 11). Normal age-related memory decline mainly affects the ability to take in new information. Another ability that seems to be particularly vulnerable to ageing is the ability to remember the source of new information and details about the context in which you heard it. This difficulty is thought to be responsible for some of the repetition in conversation that increases in old age.

Mild cognitive impairment

Mild cognitive impairment (MCI) is the name given to memory difficulties that are beyond those associated with normal age-related decline but are not significant enough to interfere with an individual's daily activities. There are a number of different reasons for MCI, many of which are described in this book, but in elderly people MCI is often a precursor to the onset of dementia. People who have additional difficulties in domains other than memory may be more likely to develop dementia than those with difficulties limited to memory. In some cases MCI remains stable over time and may just represent an extreme of normal age-related decline. When MCI is due to depression or anxiety and the underlying problem is treated, the symptoms can often resolve.

MRI scans often show loss of the grey matter in the brains of people with MCI. This tends to occur along a continuum, with mild grey matter loss associated with MCI and more extensive loss seen in Alzheimer's Disease. There are currently no proven treatments for MCI, although some studies have reported that people with MCI who regularly take folic acid and Vitamin B12 supplements are less likely to go on to develop Alzheimer's Disease than those who don't take the supplements. These vitamins are known to inhibit the production of an amino acid called homocysteine, and high levels of homocysteine in the bloodstream have been associated with an increased risk of dementia, so there may be something in it. The benefits of these supplements have yet to be proved with a randomized controlled clinical trial but, as with the blueberries discussed in Chapter 10, there is little to lose by adding these vitamins to your diet and potentially much to gain.

Use it or lose it?

In physical health it is clear that the more you use your body, the fitter it becomes. When people are ill and bedridden, their muscles can begin to waste away after just a few days. Similarly, astronauts on the Space Station experience measureable muscle wastage after just 72 hours of weightlessness. Constant use of the muscles maintains a healthy blood flow and ensures that plenty of oxygen gets to the tissue to keep it healthy. But can the same be said for the brain? Lifestyles that incorporate lots of mental stimulation, so-called 'cognitively active lifestyles', have been the subject of much research in recent years. There is plenty of evidence that people who lead a cognitively active lifestyle have a lower risk of memory problems in old age, but this could just as easily be a consequence as a cause. After all, one of the earliest features of a progressive decline in memory function is the 'I just can't be bothered with it' feeling that mentally challenging activities generate. It makes sense that a lack of engagement with mentally challenging activities may be caused directly by underlying brain pathology. However, it is also possible that the clear associations between preserved memory function and a cognitively active lifestyle might be due to the fact that mental stimulation slows down memory decline by creating some kind of mental reserve. It's a chicken-and-egg conundrum that researchers have been working hard to solve. In 2013, researchers from Rush University in Chicago came one step closer to solving the puzzle.

Keeping dementia at bay

Researchers from Chicago have been following over 1,500 people over the age of 55 since 1997. The participants in the study undergo regular memory tests and have completed numerous questionnaires about their lives over the past 16 years and counting. The researchers asked the participants how often they read books, wrote letters and sought out new information as a child, as a young adult and in middle age. They found that being cognitively active in both early and later life was associated with better performance on memory tests when the people reached old age. The researchers found that, compared to average rates of age-related decline, memory skills declined 42 per cent faster for participants who rarely read and wrote early in life and 32 per cent slower for those who had been very cognitively active from a young age.

There is also a lot of evidence that people who maintain an active social life tend to have fewer memory complaints than those who become isolated as they become older.

So, can you do anything to slow down the inevitable decline in memory skills as you get older? The answer seems to be 'yes'. Read more books, play more games, complete puzzles and stay socially active. Keeping your brain stimulated shouldn't be a chore; no one is suggesting you go back to school, but seek out something you enjoy, something that makes you think, and make sure that you find time for it on a regular basis. Learning a new skill seems to be a particularly effective strategy. One study found that learning to juggle increased brain volumes. For many people in full-time employment, their work more than meets their requirements in this area. It is therefore particularly important for people to think about how they will maintain adequate levels of mental stimulation as they approach retirement. The University of the Third Age (U3A) is a fantastic resource for older people who are no longer in full-time work but are still looking for a mental challenge. It provides opportunities for members to pursue learning, not for qualifications but for fun (see 'Useful addresses and resources', page 116, for more information).

13

Amnesia

'Amnesia', from the Greek *a*, meaning 'without', and *mnesia*, 'memory', refers to a total absence of memory. Short periods of amnesia occur when the brain is unable to process new information properly for some reason, usually through illness, injury, chemical imbalance or, very rarely, severe psychological trauma.

Neurological conditions

Many neurological conditions can lead to short periods of amnesia. People with epilepsy are often amnesic for the events that occur during their seizures; if they have generalized tonic clonic seizures (the fall-to-the-ground, violent shaking kind) they are always amnesic for the event. During these kinds of seizures, normal brain activity is disrupted so incoming information can't be processed properly. It's not a case that the memories are somehow 'locked' inside the brain; new information is not processed and so cannot ever be recalled later. Sometimes it can take a while for the brain to recover from a big seizure and the period of amnesia associated with the attack can extend a few hours afterwards. Doctors call this the post-ictal period ('post' = 'after', 'ictal' = 'seizure'). Although many people with epilepsy can be troubled with memory problems on days when they don't experience any seizures, this pure form of amnesia tends to be limited to the events that occur immediately before, during and after a seizure.

There is, however, a rare kind of epilepsy, called transient epileptic amnesia (TEA), where the only manifestation that something is wrong is that the individual is suddenly unable to remember things that have happened in the past. This may include recent events from the past couple of weeks or events from much further back. People with this condition also find it very difficult to retain any new information that is given to them while the attack is going on, but they can carry on conversations and continue with routine activities. In one famous case reported in the medical literature, one man managed to complete a game of golf during one of these attacks. Although big gaps open up and people are unable to retrieve large chunks of information from the past during these attacks, they nevertheless know who they are and tend to know those around them. Doctors still don't know much about this unusual condition, but it seems that there is some abnormal activity in the part of the brain that consolidates memory which temporarily prevents any new memories forming for a few hours. It tends to affect people in their early sixties and affects more men than women. The attacks tend to occur in the morning and generally last less than an hour, although there are some rare cases where the amnesia has persisted for days. This is currently thought to be a very rare kind of epilepsy, although researchers who work in the area think that it is probably underdiagnosed and may be more common than the current statistics suggest.

People who experience severe head injuries also have periods of amnesia where they cannot remember the events prior to and after the impact that caused the injury. Generally speaking, the length of the amnesia correlates with the severity of the head injury, so much so that doctors routinely use the duration of post-traumatic amnesia (PTA) to assess the severity of the head injury the patient has sustained. PTA is the length of time it takes until someone who has had a head injury is able to start remembering things on a continual basis again. This is often long after the patient recovers consciousness, and in very severe cases it can last months. In very severe head injuries, people are sometimes unable to remember the events that led up to the accident. This is called retrograde amnesia. Like people with epilepsy, people who survive head injuries often experience significant memory problems once they recover.

More rarely, the brain's capacity to process new information can be permanently damaged. Anterograde amnesia is a condition where someone is completely unable to form any new memories at all. If the brain's processing centres become irrevocably damaged, nothing ever gets processed deeply enough to be remembered later. People with very profound anterograde amnesia live in a permanent 'present'. They are unable to recall what happened even 30 minutes previously. Generally their memory for events that happened prior to the onset of the amnesia remains intact, so they can remember their name and autobiographical information. They also retain the abilities to talk, read, play the piano, ride a bike, etc. Basically, any information that they learnt prior to the onset of the amnesia is still there but they cannot learn anything new.

Henry Molaison (H.M.), 1926–2006

Henry Molaison was a 27-year-old Canadian manual worker in 1953 when he underwent a new experimental surgery for his epilepsy. Henry's surgeon removed both his right and left hippocampi in an attempt to cure his epilepsy. The surgery was successful in stopping his seizures but Henry paid a dreadful price. From the day of the surgery until the day he died, 53 years later, he had a dense amnesia and was unable to learn any new information at all. It's as if his life was stuck in 1953. His dense amnesia was the subject of over 500 scientific studies of memory and taught us much about the critical brain structures needed for memory.

Although a number of very different conditions can lead to anterograde amnesia, they are all fortunately quite rare. Most are associated with a fairly sudden onset of problems. Anterograde amnesia can develop after infection with the herpes simplex virus if the patient develops encephalitis. Infection with the herpes simplex virus is very common in the general population, with the most frequent manifestation being cold sores around the mouth. Once someone is infected the virus never leaves the body, but that is not usually a problem as the body produces antibodies which prevent the spread of the virus to other sites. It may mean that cold sores recur from time to time, but as anyone who suffers from them knows they tend to come back at the same place each time. Very rarely, the virus reactivates and transmits itself along the nerve cells to the brain, where it seems to have a preference for the temporal lobes, the key structures in the brain for memory. If this happens, the patient develops encephalitis – an inflammation of the brain. This is a very serious condition: left untreated, two out of three people will die. Even when it is treated, the majority of survivors are left with severe neurological problems including profound memory difficulties.

The brain damage caused by some kinds of stroke can also lead to the development of a severe anterograde amnesia, particularly if the blood supply in the middle cerebral artery – the artery that transports vital oxygen to the temporal lobes – is interrupted. Some cases of amnesia have been reported in people with epilepsy after they have experienced status epilepticus – a very prolonged seizure that would not stop.

Sometimes the onset of the amnesia is more gradual. In Korsakoff's Syndrome, brain damage occurs over an extended period of time in people with a long history of alcohol abuse; eventually it can lead to an inability to process new information and the development of amnesia. People with Korsakoff's Syndrome have difficulties learning new information and recalling recent events. Sometimes large gaps in their memories for events from the past also open up. Although their memory problems are very severe, their social skills and problem-solving abilities are relatively unaffected. Thus, people with Korsakoff's Syndrome may be able to carry on a coherent conversation without difficulty. However, minutes afterwards they will be unable to remember any of it, or even that a conversation took place at all. A common way of coping with these gaping holes in memory is to fill in the gaps with likely scenarios. This is called confabulation. People with Korsakoff's Syndrome aren't being deliberately deceitful when they do this: they often actually believe their invented explanations. A dense amnesia persists in about 25 per cent of cases, even after treatment. About half of those who develop the syndrome improve following treatment if they are able to give up alcohol, but most are left with some everyday memory problems.

Although people often use the term 'Alzheimer's' to refer to dementia, there are actually many different types of dementia of which Alzheimer's is just one (see Chapter 14). In the majority of dementias, the lack of ability to make new memories is one of the first things that sufferers (and their relatives) notice, although specialist testing often reveals other difficulties in problem-solving and using words too. As the disease progresses, access to the long-term store of memories can also become affected, and cognitive problems begin to extend beyond memory. In the late stages of dementia the person often develops anterograde and retrograde amnesia, the inability to remember new information and the inability to retrieve established memories from the past. See Chapter 14 for a more detailed discussion of the memory and other cognitive difficulties associated with dementia and ways of coping with these problems.

Psychogenic amnesia

'Psychogenic amnesia' refers to a very rare psychological condition where people suddenly forget all their autobiographical details. They normally come to the notice of the authorities when they are found confused and wandering, or on public transport, and are unable to give their name or address or any details about their previous lives. It is often difficult to discover their true identity as these people tend to be found without any identifying information on them like a wallet or mobile phone. When they are finally reunited with their loved ones, they do not recognize them or anything about their previous lives. All medical investigations are normal in these people. In particular, their brain scans do not show any damage or disease: nothing to account for such a catastrophic collapse in memory. This kind of memory loss often afflicts fictional characters in the movies, but in reality there have only been a handful of cases of psychogenic amnesia presented in the medical literature. Doctors still have much to learn about this rare condition, but the information we have to date suggests that it may be an extreme psychological response to a desire to change key aspects of a life and to start again.

Unknown White Male

On 2 July 2003 Doug Bruce, a 37-year-old wealthy British stockbroker, left his New York apartment at about 8 p.m. Twelve hours later he found himself on the subway with no idea who he was and nothing to identify him. Doctors were unable to find any physical cause for the amnesia. Doug started recording his 're-entry' into his world just one week after the onset of his amnesia. Not only did he not recognize his friends and his family, but he had forgotten the tastes of familiar food, what it felt like to swim in the sea and what rain looked and felt like. Yet he was able to talk and read and write, and could hold his own in conversations about Middle Eastern politics. Two years later, he released a controversial film, called *Unknown White Male*, about his experience. While some people think he is a medical mystery, others think the whole thing is a hoax, pointing out several inconsistencies in the incredible story, medical and otherwise. See 'Useful addresss and resources', page 116, to read more about this controversial case.

The Hollywood treatment

Unlike in real life, where identity is rather robust and only really disappears in people with advanced brain disease or severe psychiatric disturbance, loss of identity is commonplace in movie characters. However, they generally don't have the significant everyday memory difficulties that tend to accompany such a catastrophic loss, and indeed many fictional characters manage to both create and maintain entirely new lives shortly after their identity is erased from their minds. Screenwriters have exploited the dramatic possibilities of this kind of amnesia since the dawn of cinema. In *The Matrimonial Bed* (1930), one of the earliest talking movies ever made, a wealthy landowner starts a new life as a hairdresser, complete with a new wife, after he develops amnesia brought on by a train crash. Trained assassins seem to have an unfortunate tendency to forget their vocation, and in both *The Bourne Identity* (2002) and *The Long Kiss Goodnight* (1996) the hunter becomes the prey following the onset of amnesia. A different perspective is taken in the amusing parody *The Bourne Identity Crisis* (2003) where the lead character forgets that he is gay and becomes convinced that he is a trained assassin instead! While these scenarios are neurologically improbable, some amnesic syndromes in the movies bear no relation whatsoever to any authentic neurological or psychiatric conditions. In *50 First Dates* (2004) Drew Barrymore has no difficulties in laying down new memories each day, but her memories are obliterated by sleep every night. This idea is turned on its head in *Groundhog Day* (1993), where it is only the hero who retains any recall of the previous day's events, while the rest of the world suffers a collective and global amnesia, perpetually reliving the same day without any recollection at all.

Coping with amnesia

Since amnesia usually results from irreversible brain damage, ways of coping with it usually focus on establishing set routines and consistency in the individual's environment. This aids implicit memory. Implicit memory is knowledge that we may not be conscious of, but that guides our behaviour nevertheless. In a famous psychology experiment, a doctor greeted an amnesic patient with a handshake when they first met. The doctor had a device strapped to his palm that gave the patient a small electric shock when they shook hands, the kind of device that is sold in joke shops. When the doctor met the patient again the following day, the patient had no recall of their previous meeting or of ever seeing the doctor before, but he was nevertheless reluctant to shake hands, although he could not say why. The mild shock and pain of the first contact had bypassed the broken memory system and created an implicit memory.

Establishing set routines can help to establish implicit memories in amnesic patients. With much repetition, people can sometimes be 'trained' to instinctively check a calendar every morning or in response to set cues such as mealtimes. Portable digital devices (such as tablet computers and smartphones) can also be sometimes used to set reminders and to store key pieces of information for people with amnesia, increasing their independence and reducing the burden on carers. These strategies are more effective in people with stable amnesia, rather than those with a progressive condition.

Although amnesia can have a profound impact on someone's ability to socialize, it is important to ensure that people with amnesia do not become socially isolated. Discussing events from the past, for which the amnesic person may have intact recollections, can ensure mutually satisfying contact for both amnesics and their carers. A number of support groups and on-line forums are available for people who care for those with amnesia. Further information can be found in 'Useful addresses and resources' at the back of this book.

Summary

Fortunately, true amnesia is rare, but when it does occur it has a devastating impact on the individual and his or her loved ones. In some cases the period of amnesia is short-lived and limited. In other conditions the length of amnesia expands as disease progresses. There is normally nothing that can be done to 'restore' memories that should have been processed during a temporary period of amnesia (such as during an epileptic seizure or following a head injury). The information just isn't there. In other neurological conditions, such as the amnesic syndrome that can develop after some forms of encephalitis, the mechanism for encoding new memories has been irrevocably damaged. In dementia the mechanisms for encoding new information and those for retrieving old information are slowly eroded as the disease progresses. Strategies for dealing with this kind of memory loss are limited and are generally restricted to environmental adaptations to ensure as familiar an environment as possible for the person and education for loved ones to help them understand the condition and the impact it has.

14

When to seek further help

Sometimes memory problems are a symptom of something more serious than just normal ageing. This chapter discusses some of the tell-tale memory problems that indicate something more worrying may be going on and has some suggestions for when it may be helpful to check things out with a doctor.

Although people often use the term 'Alzheimer's Disease' as a catch-all term for dementia, Alzheimer's Disease is actually just one of many different types of progressive brain disease. All dementias involve a progressive deterioration and loss of brain function. This loss is irreversible and at present unstoppable, although there are a number of new drugs available that may slow down the process in some cases. Different types of dementias can be characterized by the order in which different brain regions and functions become affected. They can also be distinguished from each other by the different processes that are causing the brain cells to die.

Alzheimer's Disease

The reason that 'Alzheimer's Disease' has become a popular short-hand to describe all dementias is that it is the most common form of dementia. It accounts for approximately 70 per cent of all cases of dementia in the UK. Most people who develop Alzheimer's Disease are over the age of 65. The risk of getting Alzheimer's Disease doubles every five years after the age of 65. Nearly 50 per cent of people over the age of 85 have the disease.

The history of Alzheimer's Disease

In 1907 Dr Alois Alzheimer presented the autopsy results of a 56-year-old women at a psychiatry meeting in a Munich hospital. He published his talk a year later. Before her death the woman had

had a five-year history of cognitive and language problems, auditory hallucinations, delusions, paranoia and aggressive behaviour. At the autopsy, Alzheimer discovered plaques, tangles (types of protein deposit) and arteriosclerotic changes in her brain. All these markers were well known to be associated with dementia at the time, so how did Alzheimer's name become so inextricably linked with the condition? Medical historians think his original intention wasn't to describe a new disease at all, but rather to point out that senile dementia could occur in younger people as well as the elderly. However, his head of department wrote a textbook the following year proclaiming 'Alzheimer's Disease' as a new disease. He based these claims on just two cases: the original case and a second mysterious case, who historians now believe was actually the same woman with her name and other minor features changed. It transpired that the academic department in which Alzheimer worked was under great pressure to discover new diseases. Their research funding depended on it. Although a number of other scientists across the world pointed out at the time that nothing that Alzheimer had presented was new, a series of political and sociological circumstances meant that the name stuck. Given this history, it's ironic that the term 'Alzheimer's Disease' now refers to the typical form of dementia that occurs in old age.

In Alzheimer's Disease, the parts of the brain that process new information and commit it to memory are usually the first to malfunction. As the disease begins to manifest itself, people with Alzheimer's Disease often have significant difficulties remembering people's names and find it difficult to recall recent events. Apathy and low mood can also be early symptoms. Although memory problems are often the first overt symptom that something is wrong, the process may have started many years earlier. In the early stages of the disease, these memory difficulties can be mild and many people are able to continue to live independently; however, as the disease progresses, people begin to forget things from their own personal history and lose the ability to perform challenging mental tasks – for example, counting backwards from 100 by 7 each time. Eventually the gaps in memory and thinking become very noticeable. People may no longer be able to recall their current address or phone number and may give information from their past instead, such as their childhood address. At this stage they may also begin to lose very well-rehearsed information. They often lose track of the days of the week and where they are, particularly if they are presented with new surroundings. At this stage they can usually still recall significant details about themselves and close family members, and can feed and toilet themselves. In the final stages of the disease people lose the ability to respond to their environment and are no longer able to speak, although they may still say words or phrases. They lose the ability to control movement and eventually swallowing becomes impaired.

It often takes many years after the onset of this process before anyone notices that something is wrong. However, once memory problems have been established they tend to progress fairly steadily.

In people with advanced Alzheimer's Disease, scans often show that the brain has shrunk, and areas associated with memory are particularly small. Other features include the presence of plaques and tangles that are hallmarks of the disease.

Vascular dementia

The second most common dementia in the UK is vascular dementia. It is sometimes also called multi infarct dementia. Vascular dementia occurs when the arteries supplying the brain burst or become blocked, starving parts of the brain of oxygen. Vascular dementia is the result of lots of small stokes. Each one leaves part of the brain damaged irrevocably. Over time, larger and larger regions of the brain become damaged and die. People with vascular dementia often have a history of larger strokes too. The risks associated with vascular dementia are exactly the same as those associated with heart disease. High blood pressure, obesity, a sedentary lifestyle, smoking and a family history of vascular disease (cerebral or cardiac) are all associated with a higher risk of developing vascular dementia in older age. While the risk of vascular dementia more than doubles in those with a history of alcohol abuse, consumption of one to six drinks weekly is associated with a lower risk of dementia among older adults, compared to total abstention. As far as alcohol is concerned, it seems that a little of what you fancy may do you good, but moderation is the key.

Vascular dementias present in many different ways. It very much depends on which part of the brain each stroke damages as to how that will manifest itself in someone's behaviour or thinking. As with Alzheimer's Disease, memory functions can often be affected, but other features such as hallucinations or the ability to coordinate fine motor movements can also be compromised. If the regions at the front of the brain are affected, people may demonstrate impaired judgement or become rather disinhibited. They may make inappropriate or hurtful comments to their friends and family. They may not always realize that they have upset someone, or understand why someone would be hurt by what they have said. They may lose the ability to plan properly. People with vascular dementia often have a characteristic appearance on their brain scans with lots of white speckles and dots representing each mini stroke. Vascular dementias can often be differentiated from other forms of dementia by the 'stepwise' nature of the loss of function. People may find that they (or their loved ones with the disease) suddenly can't do something that they could manage the day before, or that a new symptom suddenly appears. In other forms of dementia these losses tend to be more gradual and it is more difficult to pinpoint exactly when someone lost the ability to carry out a specific task. As with Alzheimer's Disease, there are a number of things that can be attempted to try to slow the progress of vascular dementia, including controlling blood pressure and using statins to try to improve vascular health. However, it is a sad fact that once a vascular dementia starts, the cerebral arteries are already too damaged to reverse the process. The most effective preventions for vascular dementia, like those for heart disease, need to be implemented in childhood and maintained throughout adulthood.

Other forms of dementia

Other less common forms of dementia include Lewy Body Disease, frontotemporal dementia and mixed dementias.

Lewy bodies are abnormal clumps of a specific protein called alpha-synuclein that develop in the grey matter of the brain. Alpha-synuclein is the protein that builds up in the brains of people with Parkinson's Disease (PD), but in PD the clumps initially develop in deeper parts of the brain and primarily affect movement. People with Lewy body dementia often experience memory problems but also tend to have sleep disturbances, hallucinations and difficulties with motor coordination in the early stages of the disease, unlike those with Alzheimer's Disease.

In frontotemporal dementia, areas at the front and side of the brain are particularly affected. Rather than memory problems, initial symptoms may include personality changes and difficulties with language. There may be marked word-finding difficulties or difficulties in understanding what someone else is saying. The progression of the disease in frontotemporal dementia is generally more rapid than that seen in Alzheimer's Disease and people seem to develop it at a slightly younger age, at around 60. Frontotemporal dementia is normally diagnosed on the basis of the pattern of deterioration, rather than any hallmark characteristics on a brain scan.

Although these different types of dementia have certain characteristic patterns in the early and later stages, there is a large degree of overlap. Everybody's presentation is different and it is often not easy to distinguish one type of dementia from another, particularly in the early stages. Some people develop multiple types of dementia. Signs of both Alzheimer's Disease and vascular dementia are not uncommon on the brain scans of people with dementia, and Lewy bodies can also be often identified. Recent brain imaging studies have suggested that these mixed dementias are more common than previously thought.

When to seek help

In an increasingly ageing population, dementia is a frightening prospect for both ourselves and our loved ones. The Alzheimer's Association has devised a simple checklist of ten features that *may* indicate difficulties over and above those that would be expected given normal aged-related changes in function.

Memory difficulties that are disrupting your life

The first relates to the extent to which the memory difficulties disrupt your life. It is entirely normal to sometimes forget people's names or to put the kettle on and walk away. This tends to happen when we are busy and distracted by other things. The information is not lost and we tend to remember it later on. But if your memory problems are beginning to disrupt your life, to the extent that you need to ask for the same information over and over again, or that, without family members to help you, you just can't remember what you need to do each day, then there may be a problem. It's perfectly OK to rely on a diary or calendar to remind you of appointments, but if you rely on them to the extent that it is the only way you have any idea of what you should be doing each day, again there may be a problem. Written notes should prompt your memory. The contents should not come as a surprise each time you look, and you should not have to look over and over again. As a very general rule of thumb, if you think, 'Aah, yes!' when you see something scheduled on the calendar there isn't a problem; if written reminders frequently don't ring any bells at all, something more than just normal age-related decline may be going on.

Deterioration in other cognitive processes

Although people tend to focus on memory difficulties when they are worried about dementia, it's important to recognize that many types of dementia affect other cognitive processes too. Some people find it very difficult to plan relatively simple tasks, like cooking a meal, or solve logistical problems, particularly if there are a number of steps involved. Sometimes they just don't know where to start. This can lead to a gradual 'putting off' of tasks that then begin to build up over time. Sometimes people are able to make a start but then get lost mid-task. Sometimes people are able to complete these tasks but they take much, much longer than they should and the individual needs to check and recheck to make sure that things are right. It's completely normal to make occasional mistakes and to find it difficult to focus your concentration when your mind is preoccupied with other things. It's OK to boil the kettle a few times before you get round to making a cup of tea and even to overcook the odd meal, but if you find that these things are happening more and more often and that even simple tasks require a huge mental effort and energy you don't seem to have, there may be a problem.

Emily's story
Dad had always dealt with the household bills and paperwork for the 50 years that he'd been married to Mum. In his early seventies he began to get a bit forgetful and started to repeat himself and we all joked about dementia, including him. No one really thought it was happening. It was only when Mum had a fall and went into the hospital, and I moved in for a couple of weeks to help out, that I realized how he had been struggling. All of the household paperwork was in disarray and they were about to be disconnected from the electricity. It was heart-breaking to be in the study, which had always been such an ordered, efficient space. Everything was in such disorder and Dad didn't have a clue where to start.

Increasing difficulty with familiar tasks

One of the most obvious signs that something is wrong in someone with dementia is an increasing difficulty in being able to carry out familiar, routine tasks. These can be domestic chores or leisure activities. Other worrying signs may be difficulties driving to familiar locations and periods of disorientation while out and about. While these features may be worrying, it's perfectly OK to need help getting to grips with all the new technologies that are now part of everyday life (mobile phones, computers and the internet, complicated remote controls for satellite TVs, etc.) and there is no need to worry if you need to be shown how these things work a few times before they become a help rather than a hindrance in your life.

Lillian and Matthew
Lillian, a retired school teacher, regularly came to the clinic with her husband Matthew, who had been diagnosed with Alzheimer's Disease two years earlier. Three years prior to the onset of any obvious difficulties, the couple had had to withdraw from the bridge club as Matthew was unable to play the game and appeared to just 'forget' the rules. At the time Lillian had attributed their withdrawal to other changes in their lives, but in retrospect she realized that this was probably the onset of her husband's difficulties.

Being unable to keep track of time

People with Alzheimer's Disease can lose track of time. Sometimes they find it difficult to remember the exact date or the day of the week. In later stages of the condition people can lose track of the seasons or the time of day and their sleep–wake patterns can be disrupted as a result. However, there is nothing to worry about if you occasionally get the wrong day or are a couple of days out with the date. Temporary difficulties in keeping track of the days of the week and the exact date often happen when people first retire and they lose the previously rigid structure to the week imposed by work. It can also happen when people move into new environments, such as sheltered accommodation. Any life changes that result in one day being much like another can result in difficulties keeping track of time, until a new routine is established. However, if you find that you frequently don't know the date or the day of the week and can't figure it out, it may be a sign that something is wrong.

Difficulties with interpreting visual images or spatial awareness

As we get older our eyesight changes. These changes begin in our early forties, when most people develop a degree of long-sightedness and start to need glasses to read small text. These changes continue into older age and cataracts are common post-retirement. One study found that 40 per cent of people aged between 70 and 80 had developed cataracts, while nearly 70 per cent of people over the age of 80 were affected. Glaucoma is the second leading cause of blindness and its prevalence also increases dramatically with age. It affects about one in 200 people under the age of 50 but more than one in ten people over the age of 80. The loss of vision in glaucoma often occurs very gradually over a long period of time. It is unsurprising, then, that many older people report difficulties with vision. However, difficulties making sense of visual images and problems in working out spatial relationships between objects may be a sign of dementia. These include problems in interpreting written text (difficulties that are not due to reduced acuity) and difficulties judging distances. These problems often come to the fore when driving at dusk, when people may find that they misjudge the speed of other vehicles or may miss unexpected obstacles altogether.

Jennifer's story
When driving back from a visit to her daughter's house, Jennifer drove her car straight into a large hole in the middle of some road works, writing the vehicle off in the process. She was adamant that the hole and the road works were unmarked and that the barricades that should

have been around the hole were by the side of the road. She com-
plained to the council. A subsequent investigation revealed that Jennifer
had driven over a road sign and through the bollards and warning tape
before she had ended up in the large hole.

Deteriorating judgement and bizarre decision-making

It's not just spatial judgements that can become progressively
inaccurate in dementia. Poor judgements in everyday life can
also develop and people can begin to make uncharacteristically
bizarre, impulsive or ill-thought-out decisions. These decisions
often involve financial transactions and unfortunately criminals are
all too aware of this. Some deliberately target elderly people, hoping
to exploit this weakness with improbable scams that most people
would see through quite easily.

Helen: finding love and lies on-line
There is nothing new about charming conmen smooth-talking their way
into people's lives and their bank accounts. But with the advent of the
internet, conmen don't need to be smooth, charming (or even men!)
to steal from their victims, since the scam is conducted entirely on-line
under an assumed cyber-identity. Helen, a solicitor in her late fifties, had
been widowed for four years when, unbeknown to her children, she
signed up to a dating site. She quickly established an on-line relationship with Robert, a recent widower in the adjacent county who shared
all her interests. Although they made plans to meet, it was always called
off at the last minute. It didn't take long for Robert to start asking for
money – for car repairs, theatre tickets, all kinds of things to facilitate
their meeting, but something always came up at the last minute to stop
them getting together. In the space of six months Helen transferred over
£15,000 to her on-line lover. It was only after she had exhausted her
resources and asked her children for a loan that they realized something
was wrong. Helen's daughter, Kirsty, said, 'We couldn't believe it when
we read the emails. The spelling mistakes and inconsistencies were rife.
Mum has always had such a clear, legal mind. Dad worked for a while
in the victim support unit and they used to discuss exactly these kinds
of cases. She would never have been fooled by such a clumsy amateur
scam in her right mind.'

Falling for a dating scam, or any other kind, is not a sign of
dementia. It can happen to anyone at any age. The fraudsters are
often clever and know how exactly how to reel in their victims in

a sophisticated, drawn-out process. But a failure to spot obvious deceptions or clearly flawed plans can be a red flag that something is wrong, particularly if, as in Helen's case, you know that you or your loved one would have ordinarily seen the flaws a mile off.

Increasing difficulty with words

As discussed in Chapter 6, word-finding difficulties are very common indeed and are one of the most frustrating memory difficulties that people report. Sometimes people seem to have a 'block' on the same word over and over again. For others, word-finding difficulties strike most often when they are in social situations and have had a glass of wine or two. These difficulties are a normal part of age-related decline and can begin as early as the fourth decade of life. In dementia, people begin to develop new problems using words. They may call things by the wrong name, for example calling a 'pen' an 'ink write' or a watch an 'arm time'. They may also develop more general problems with conversation. These can include trouble following the thread of a conversation. Sometimes they fail to follow normal conversational rules and can cut across other people or contribute ideas that don't seem to follow on from what's been said before. People with dementia sometimes stop mid-flow in a conversation and have no idea what they were going to say or what they were talking about. It is common for people to sometimes repeat stories and anecdotes to their friends and family, but if this repetition happens when someone has just told the same story, minutes before, it may be a sign of something more than just a 'senior moment'.

Losing things and being unable to retrace your steps

The Transport for London Lost Property Office is testament to the fact that everybody loses things sometimes, even important things. The office collects and collates over 150,000 items left each year in the tubes, trains, buses and black taxi cabs of London. It is easy to understand how people can leave their scarfs, umbrellas and perhaps handbags behind. However, the considerable cache of false teeth, wheelchairs, pushchairs and crutches that are handed in every week suggests that a trip on the tube is akin to a visit to

Lourdes for some. A wedding dress, a coffin and a set of breast implants en route to Harley Street have also turned up at the office. Losing things is part of everyday life. We are taught two rules as children to minimize our seemingly innate tendency to lose things. The first is to have a clear 'home' for everything, be it hooks for keys or a drawer for cutlery. If everything has its place we are more likely to automatically put it back where it belongs. This doesn't always happen, of course, but when it doesn't, the second rule kicks in . . . retrace your steps to where you last saw it. If nobody has disturbed the scene, this usually results in the lost object being found. Losing things occasionally and retracing your steps to find them is entirely normal. However, losing things and not being able to retrace your steps, or frequently finding things in odd places (a phone in the fridge, cheese in a drawer) may be a sign that something is wrong. The frequent loss of objects can become very confusing for people and sometimes leads to the development of paranoia and the sense that other people must be to blame for the losses and the seemingly inexplicable places where things may turn up.

Withdrawal from social activities

Somebody with dementia may start to withdraw from social activities. This is often due to the difficulties that have been described above, including trouble in following conversations, loss of confidence in driving and difficulties in making plans. Memory difficulties prompted Lillian's husband to withdraw from the bridge club, two years before he was diagnosed with Alzheimer's Disease. It is entirely normal to feel weary of work, family or social obligations sometimes, but if this is a new and pervasive feeling, something may be wrong. Changes in this arena don't necessarily signal the onset of Alzheimer's Disease. They are also seen in depression. This is why depression will be one of the diagnoses that a doctor will want to rule out before diagnosing Alzheimer's Disease . As with the other signs, the key word here is 'change'. If someone has always found social obligations trying then a failure to engage in older age is not a worrying sign. However, if someone noticeably withdraws from activities he or she has previously enjoyed, something may be wrong and a trip to the GP may help to identify what it is.

Changes in mood and personality

It is unsurprising that, with all these changes, the personalities of people with Alzheimer's Disease can alter. Previously easy-going, gentle people may become blunt, suspicious, fearful or anxious. These reactions are often more pronounced when people are in unfamiliar places or situations. This is different from becoming 'set in your ways' and liking things to be done in a particular way. It is completely normal to be irritated when people don't respect this or try to impose their own routines on you, particularly when this is in your own home.

Summary

This chapter has summarized some of the key features that may indicate the onset of Alzheimer's Disease or other forms of dementia. The list is not exhaustive and different people may exhibit different combinations of symptoms. In the early stages of the disease it is often not an either–or situation with respect to these symptoms; rather, they exist along a continuum. Everybody experiences some of these problems some of the time. However, if a lot of these problems are happening on a regular basis it's worth making an appointment with the GP to get yourself checked out. Making a checklist based on these ten signs might be helpful to guide the discussion, and it is also useful to take someone along with you. There are a number of other conditions that the GP will want to exclude before a diagnosis of suspected dementia will be given. If dementia does seem to be the probable diagnosis the GP may be able to offer medication on a palliative basis, but more importantly he or she will be able to tell you about the support services that are available to help you through diagnosis and beyond.

15

Conclusions

There are five stages in coping with memory problems.

Understand how memory works

The first stage is learning how memory works to gain an appreciation of what is normal and what is not. Realizing that memory is fallible, malleable and unreliable, even in the best of circumstances, helps to ensure that we have realistic expectations of our memory (and that of other people). Some age-related decline in memory function is as inevitable as the physical changes associated with age. No matter how fit and healthy they are, 50-year-olds do not have the bodies of 20-year-olds. The same can be said for our brains. If you are troubled by memory failures, keep a diary or log of the situations you have trouble with to help you get to know what makes things better or worse. There may be a pattern related to the time of day, hunger or fatigue when these problems are more likely to occur. Does it help to rest, take a walk or have a snack? Understanding how memory works will help you to understand where it is going wrong when you experience memory problems.

Maximize the health of your hippocampi

Your hippocampi are two of the most precious assets you have when it comes to preserving memory function. Look after them. They are particularly vulnerable to the damaging effects of a diverse range of medical conditions including cardiovascular disease, atrial fibrillation, diabetes, high blood pressure and obesity, particularly if excess fat is carried around the middle as opposed to the hips and thighs. All of the well-established medical advice regarding cardiovascular fitness will benefit hippocampal health (see 'Useful addresses and resources', page 115, for sources of advice for looking after your heart). Other treatable conditions associated with hippocampal damage include obstructive sleep apnoea, Vitamin B12 deficiency and clinical depression.

The hippocampal damage associated with all these conditions is a risk factor for conversion from the normal ageing process to developing mild cognitive impairment and dementia. Fortunately, lifestyle changes can have a significant positive impact on hippocampal health. Research has found that regular physical exercise, dietary changes, cognitive stimulation and optimal treatment of underlying medical conditions can slow down or even reverse age-related shrinkage in the hippocampi.

Maximize your memory

There are many strategies you can use to maximize your memory capacity and minimize the nuisance of memory failures. Some are internal, self-generated strategies that ensure you encode memories as deeply as possible. These can be relatively simple strategies, such as using mnemonics to give you a 'way in' to memorized lists or saying something out loud to ensure that an automatic behaviour is consciously processed and therefore more likely to be remembered later: for example, 'It is Tuesday, I am on my way out to meet Tom for coffee and I have turned off the iron.'

In additional to these internal strategies, you can also manipulate the external environment to ease the pressure on your memory. Setting up and following fixed routines, keeping the same daily schedule and choosing a specific place for commonly lost objects and putting them there each time can all help to reduce the nuisance of common memory failures. Be aware that when you are multitasking your memory capacity will be reduced, so try to focus on one thing at a time.

Outsource memory functions

One of the most effective ways to reduce the nuisance of everyday memory problems is to remove memory from the equation and outsource the things your memory should be doing to another external medium. From the humble to-do list scrawled on the back of an envelope to the most sophisticated digital app, most of these memory aids involve writing something down in one form or another. Not only does writing something down mean that you process it more deeply, it automatically provides a clear, set record for you to consult, taking the strain from your memory. Keeping everything in one place makes it easier to find and consult your reminders. Smartphones and tablet computers allow people to keep track of multiple areas of their lives including appointments, schedules, to-do lists and important dates. Lists of useful websites, contact details, meeting notes and even books you have read or would like to read in the future can also be incorporated, with information added on the go. If these new technologies are not for you, an old-fashioned notebook and pen can do the same. However, digital apps on smartphones can come into their own when it comes to prospective memory – remembering to remember. With well-programmed alarms there is no need to remember to remember: prospective memory tasks simply become a matter of responding to a prompt. It is never too early to get into the habit of outsourcing as much as possible when it comes to taking the strain from your memory. Effective outsourcing also tends to lead to a reduction in anxiety when it comes to memory problems, which in turn improves memory function.

Know when to seek help

Sometimes memory problems are a sign of a serious neurological condition such as dementia. The older you are the more likely this is, but it is by no means inevitable, even in very old age. There is a loose pattern of memory problems that tends to be characteristic of dementia. These are outlined in Chapter 14. If, having read the descriptions of normal age-related decline and the memory problems typically seen in dementia, you are concerned about progressive deterioration, do not put off consulting your GP. Ask for an extended or double appointment to ensure that you have enough time to explain your concerns. It will be helpful if you can take a list of some of the memory problems you have noticed. Also write down any questions you may have. If possible, take a friend or family member with you to help you keep track of what is said during the consultation. If you go with someone who knows you well, he or she will also be able to give the doctor a valuable perspective on your memory problems. Your GP may be able to provide reassurance, but in the event that a dementia is suspected the doctor will be able to put you in contact with the support services you need.

Glossary

confabulation false, distorted or fabricated recollections produced without a conscious intention to deceive

encoding the basic building block and first part of the memory process that allows new information to be stored and recalled later; without adequate encoding it is impossible to recall information later on

episodic memory literally the memory for episodes or events in your past

hippocampus a seahorse-shaped part of the brain that plays a crucial role in committing new memories to the long-term store; the brain has two hippocampi (plural), one on the right-hand and one on the left-hand side of the brain

IAPT Improving Access to Psychological Therapies is a UK scheme to increase the provision of evidence-based treatments for anxiety and depression by the NHS; see <www.iapt.nhs.uk> for more details

involuntary memories vivid memories or fragments of memory that suddenly come into your mind without any conscious effort; they are usually set off by environmental triggers or cues that are processed subconsciously

mnemonic strategies techniques that help people to encode and retrieve information from memory; common mnemonics include poems, acronyms and memorable phrases

neurons brain cells that communicate with each other through electrical and chemical signals

prospective memory remembering that you need to do something at a specific point in the future; remembering to remember

sensory cues smells, tastes, sights, sounds and textures that can trigger memories; they often combine to provide triggers for memories which, although fragmentary, are rich in detail

state-dependent learning the phenomenon where memories are more easily recalled when an individual is in the same physiological or psychological state as when the memory was formed

verbal memory memory for information that is conveyed in words

visual memory memory for information that is visual (e.g. faces, landscapes and scenes)

working memory the process that allows you to hold multiple pieces of information in your mind *and* manipulate them at the same time; mental arithmetic requires working memory for success

Useful addresses and resources

Useful addresses – general (UK and USA)

Alzheimer's Association (USA)
Helpline: 1.800.272.3900 (24 hrs a day, 7 days a week)
Website: www.alz.org

Provides useful information for people in the United States, and their carers, about all kinds of dementia as well as Alzheimer's.

Alzheimer's Society (UK)
Devon House
58 St Katharine's Way
London E1W 1LB
Tel.: 020 7433 3500 (for general information, including details of other branches in the UK)
Helpline: 0300 222 11 22
Website: www.alzheimers.org.uk

The site contains a wealth of useful information for people with all forms of dementia, and their carers.

British Heart Foundation
Greater London House
180 Hampstead Road
London NW1 7AW
Tel.: 020 7935 0185 (general information)
Heart health helpline: 0300 330 3311 (9 a.m. to 5 p.m., Monday to Friday)
Website: www.bhf.org.uk

Provides advice and publishes a number of factsheets and DVDs on how to reduce cardiovascular risk. The website also hosts a chat forum for support.

Headway
Bradbury House
190 Bagnall Road
Old Basford
Nottingham NG6 8SF
Tel.: 0115 924 0800
Helpline: 0808 800 2244
Website: www.headway.org.uk

This charity provides an extensive network of groups across the UK to support people living with amnesia following a brain injury, and their carers.

National Health Service (NHS)
Website:www.nhs.uk/livewell/healthy-eating

This part of the NHS website gives sound advice on healthy eating, losing weight and superfoods. Meal planners are included, also a calculator to help you work out your Body Mass Index (BMI), and a healthy eating self-assessment tool. The online weight-loss clinic provides expert advice on losing weight, exercise and other weight-loss topics.

University of the Third Age (U3A)
19 East Street
Bromley
Kent BR1 1QE
Tel.: 020 8466 6139
Website: www.u3a.org.uk

A provider of helpful information, including details of online courses and how to find your local branch.

Finding out more about . . .

Henry Molaison
Suzanne Corkin's book *Permanent Present Tense: The unforgettable life of amnesic patient, H.M.* was published in May 2013 by Basic Books in the USA, and at the same time by Allen Lane in the UK, with the subtitle *The man with no memory, and what he taught the world.* The result is a fascinating, accessible insight into Henry's life and his legacy to neuroscience.

The Invisible Gorilla
To find out more about the gorilla experiments carried out by Professors Daniel Simons and Christopher Chabris, see www.theinvisiblegorilla. com. You can watch the videos and also take part in some of the other experiments on the site concerning attention. They have also written a book, *The Invisible Gorilla* (HarperCollins, 2010).

Unknown White Male
You can read more about this controversial case in 'A Trip Down Memory Lane' by David Segal (*Washington Post*, 22 March 2006), available to read online for free. A film on the topic, *Unknown White Male*, was made in 2006.

Stroop Test
To test yourself on the Stroop Test, visit http://faculty.washington.edu/ chudler/java/ready.html

Various resources

Anxiety
Sheldon Press publishes books on coping with anxiety; these include:

Delvin, Dr D., *How to Beat Worry and Stress* (2011)

Dryden, Dr W., *Letting Go of Anxiety and Depression* (2003)

Trickett, S., *Coping Successfully with Panic Attacks* (2009)

Drug wallet
Drug wallets are folders with plastic pockets or pill boxes with compartments to store a week's supply of medication. The idea is to stock them up once a week. By checking the box or wallet each day you can be sure that you have taken your medication. A variety of drug wallets are available on-line through Amazon (www.amazon.co.uk).

Effective study techniques and note taking
There are many guides on the internet that provide tips on how to make effective notes in lectures and meetings. Many of these are provided by universities. Some of the clearest are those from the Open University (www.open.ac.uk); this website offers skills for OU study, reading and taking notes. Full details on the PQRST, RRR and SQ3R study techniques can also be found at the website of the State College of Florida (www.scf.edu/content/PDF/ARC/How_to_study_a_reading_assignment.pdf).

Healthy diet
See **National Health Service**, page 116.

Livescribe smartpens
The livescribe pen is actually a tiny computer. It is equipped with a microphone to record what is said, a speaker for playback, a camera and a memory card. When you make notes with the pen, you can tap on the words later to hear a playback of that particular part of the recording. The livescribe system is expensive and takes some effort to master, but can be a really useful tool in study situations and formal meetings where a lot of information is presented. See www.livescribe.com/uk for more information on the system.

Living with amnesia
See **Headway**, page 115.

Memory apps
There are many memory aid apps that have been developed for both Apple and Android smartphones. The easier it is to put information in and retrieve information that has already been stored, the better. You may need to try a few before you find one that suits your style and meets your

requirements. Fortunately many are free. 'Use Your Handwriting' is a free app that allows you to 'finger write' quick notes, lists and messages and converts the scrawl into legible notes.

Index

Bold type indicates the main treatment of the topic